AIR FRYER COOKBOOK
#2020

500 Quick & Easy Air Frying Recipes that
Anyone Can Cook on a Budget
Lower Cholesterol & Shed Weight

By

WILDA BUCKLEY

a

WHAT IS AN AIR FRYER?

An air fryer is an appliance that works by circulating hot air around food to cook it by using the principle of heat convection. It has an adjustable temperature knob and timer for precise cooking.

An air fryer does not require that food be cooked in oil, hence it does not increase the fat or calorie content of the food. Constant consumption of deep-fried foods can lead to a series of medical issues such as obesity and other health problems. However, with the use of an air fryer, you can now enjoy many foods without having to worry about the side effects. With an air fryer, say no to deep-fry today.

A. Benefits of the air fryer
- Easy clean up
- Cooks food quickly
- Controls cooking time and temperature
- Versatile
- Decreases the danger of cholesterol

B. Air fryer advantages
- **Healthier Meals**

  Little to no oil is required when using an air fryer! These gadgets are perfect for making crisp French fries, onion rings, mozzarella sticks, chicken wings, and more. In contrast to a customary broiler, air frying is faster and healthier.

- **Quicker, More Efficient Cooking**

  Air fryers take only minutes to preheat, and they cook food quicker than a broiler or on the stovetop. The impact of the warm is increased by the flowing air.

  These units are more productive than a broiler. Utilizing an air fryer won't warm up your home in the summer, and the expense of the power utilized is simply pennies. Since the cooking cycle is shorter, you can see that utilizing an air fryer makes most cooking quicker and more productive!

- **Versatility**

  You can utilize air fryers to air fry, pan sear, warm, heat, cook, broil, barbecue, steam and even rotisserie in certain models. Make franks and wieners, steak, chicken bosoms or thighs, flame-broiled sandwiches, pan-seared meats, and veggies. simmered or steamed veggies, a wide range of fish and shrimp dishes, and even cakes and sweets. If your unit is large enough, you can even roast a whole chicken or turkey.

- **Space-Saving**

  Most units are about the size of an espresso machine. A few models are small and super-conservative, making them ideal for kitchenettes, apartments or RVs. An air fryer can replace a broiler and can be more helpful than a toaster oven or steamer. You will be glad to give it a home on your kitchen counter!

- **Easy to Use**

  Most fryers are extremely simple to utilize. Simply set the cooking temperature and time and put your food in the crate. Remember to shake the food occasionally during the cooking cycle, particularly for things like fries, chips, and wings. Many air fryer lovers have even trained their kids to use them to make after-school snacks!

VEGETARIAN AIR FRYER RECIPES

1. Masala Galette

INGREDIENTS

- 2 - tbsp. garam masala
- 2 - medium potatoes boiled and mashed
- 1 ½ - cup coarsely crushed peanuts
- 3 - tsp. ginger finely chopped
- 1 to 2 - tbsp. fresh coriander leaves
- 2 or 3 - green chilies finely chopped
- 1 ½ - tbsp. lemon juice
- Salt and pepper to taste

INSTRUCTIONS

1. Blend the ingredients in a bowl.
2. Form this blend into round, flat galettes.
3. Wet the galettes with a small amount of water. Coat each galette with crushed peanuts.
4. Preheat the Air Fryer to 160 F for 5 minutes.
5. Place the galettes in the fry bin and let them cook for an additional 25 minutes.
6. Continue turning them over to cook uniformly.
7. Serve with mint chutney or ketchup.

2. Potato Samosa

INGREDIENTS

For wrappers:

- 2 - tbsp. unsalted butter
- 1 ½ - cup all-purpose flour
- A pinch of salt
- Water

For filling:

- 2 to 3 - large potatoes
- ¼ - cup boiled peas
- 1 - tsp. powdered ginger
- 1 or 2 - green chilies
- ½ - tsp. cumin
- 1 - tsp. coarsely crushed coriander
- 1 - dry red chili
- A small amount of salt
- ½ - tsp. mango powder
- ½ - tsp. red chili powder.

- 1 to 2 - tbsp. coriander.

INSTRUCTIONS

1. Blend the wrapper ingredients. Let it sit while making the filling.
2. Cook the ingredients in a skillet and blend them well to make a thick paste.
3. Form the paste into balls. Cut them in half and insert the filling.
4. Preheat the Air Fryer to 300 F. Place the samosas in the fry receptacle
5. Cook for 20-25 minutes. Flip halfway through for uniform cooking.
6. Serve hot with tamarind or mint chutney.

3. Vegetable Kebab

INGREDIENTS

- 2 cups mixed vegetables
- 3 onions chopped
- 5 green chilies-roughly chopped
- 1 ½ tbsp. ginger paste
- 1 ½ tsp. garlic paste
- 1 ½ tsp. salt
- 3 tsp. lemon juice
- 2 tsp. garam masala
- 4 tbsp. chopped coriander
- 3 tbsp. cream
- 3 tbsp. chopped capsicum
- 3 eggs
- 2 ½ tbsp. white sesame seeds

INSTRUCTIONS

1. Mix the ingredients except the egg and form a smooth paste.
2. Coat the vegetables in the paste. Beat in the eggs and add salt to season.
3. Dip the vegetables in the egg mix and coat well with sesame seed.
4. Place the vegetables on skewers.
5. Preheat the Air fryer to 160 F. Cook for 25 minutes.
6. Turn the sticks over halfway through to cook uniformly.

4. Sago galette

INGREDIENTS

- 2 cup sago, soaked
- 1 ½ cup coarsely crushed peanuts
- 3 tsp. ginger finely chopped
- 1-2 tbsp. fresh coriander leaves
- 2 or 3 green chilies finely chopped
- 1 ½ tbsp. lemon juice
- Salt and pepper to taste

INSTRUCTIONS

1. Blend the ingredients in a bowl.
2. Form this blend into round, flat galettes.
3. Wet the galettes with a small amount of water. Coat each galette with crushed peanuts.
4. Preheat the Air Fryer to 160 F for 5 minutes. Place the galettes in the fry bin and let them cook for an additional 25 minutes. Continue turning them over to cook uniformly.
5. Serve with mint chutney or ketchup.

5. Stuffed Capsicum Baskets

INGREDIENTS

- For baskets:
- 3-4 long capsicum
- ½ tsp. salt
- ½ tsp. pepper powder

For filling:

- 1 medium onion
- 1 green chili
- 2 or 3 large potatoes
- 1 ½ tbsp. chopped coriander leaves
- 1 tsp. fenugreek
- 1 tsp. dried mango powder
- 1 tsp. cumin powder
- Salt and pepper

For topping:

- 3 tbsp. grated cheese
- 1 tsp. red chili flakes
- ½ tsp. oregano
- ½ tsp. basil
- ½ tsp. parsley

INSTRUCTIONS

1. Mix all of the filling ingredients in a bowl.
2. Remove the stem, seeds and top of the capsicum.
3. Sprinkle some salt and pepper inside the capsicums. Set aside.
4. Place the filling inside the peppers, leaving a little space at the top.
5. Mix topping spices and sprinkle ground cheese and seasoning on top.
6. Preheat the Air Fryer to 140 F for 5 minutes.
7. Put the capsicums in the fry case and cook for 20 minutes.

6. Macaroni Samosa

INGREDIENTS

For wrappers:
- cup all-purpose flour
- 2- tbsp. unsalted butter
- A pinch of salt to taste
- Take the amount of water sufficient

For filling:

- 3- cups boiled macaroni
- 2- onion
- 2- capsicum
- 2- Carrots
- 2- Cabbage
- 2- tbsp. soy sauce
- 2- tsp. vinegar
- 2- tbsp. ginger
- 2- tbsp. garlic
- 2- tbsp. green chilies
- 2- tbsp. ginger-garlic paste
- Some salt and pepper
- 2- tbsp. olive oil

INSTRUCTIONS

1. Blend the wrapper ingredients until smooth. Set aside while making the filling.
2. Boil the filling ingredients and blend them to make a thick paste.
3. Form the batter into balls. Cut them in half and insert the filling.
4. Preheat the Air Fryer to 300 F. Place the samosas in the fry holder and cook for 20 to 25 minutes

5. Around the midpoint, turn the samosas over for uniform cooking.
6. Serve hot with tamarind or mint chutney.

7. Burritos

INGREDIENTS

Refried beans:

- ½ cup red kidney beans
- ½ small onion
- 1 tbsp. olive oil
- 2 tbsp. tomato puree
- ¼ tsp. red chili powder
- 1 tsp. of salt
- 4-5 flour tortillas

Vegetable Filling:

- 1 tbsp. Olive oil
- 1 medium onion
- 3 flakes garlic crushed
- ½ cup French beans
- 1 cup cottage cheese
- ½ cup shredded cabbage
- 1 tbsp. coriander
- 1 tbsp. vinegar
- 1 tsp. white wine
- A pinch of salt
- ½ tsp. red chili flakes
- 1 tsp. freshly ground peppercorns
- ½ cup pickled Jalapeño s
- 2 carrots

Salad:

- 1-2 lettuce leaves shredded.
- 1 or 2 spring onions
- 1 green chili
- 1 cup of cheddar

INSTRUCTIONS

1. Cook the beans with the onion and garlic and mash them.
2. For the filling, sauté the ingredients in a pan.
3. Toss the salad ingredients together.
4. Lay the tortilla on a flat surface and place a layer of sauce and filling inside.
5. Wrap the tortilla to create a burrito.

6. Preheat the Air Fryer to 200 F. Open the fry case and place the burritos inside.
7. Cook for 15 minutes. Flip the burritos halfway through.

8. Cheese and Bean Enchiladas

INGREDIENTS

- Flour tortillas

Red sauce:

- 4 tbsp. of olive oil
- 1 ½ tsp. of garlic
- 1 ½ cups of readymade tomato puree
- 3 medium tomatoes
- 1 tsp. of sugar
- A pinch of salt
- A few red chili flakes to sprinke
- 1 tsp. of oregano

Filling:

- 2 tbsp. oil
- 2 tsp. chopped garlic
- 2 onions
- 2 capsicums
- 2 cups of readymade baked beans
- A few drops of Tabasco sauce
- 1 cup cottage cheese
- 1 cup grated cheddar
- A pinch of salt
- 1 tsp. oregano
- ½ tsp. pepper
- 1 ½ tsp. red chili flakes
- 1 tbsp. of finely chopped Jalapeño s

INSTRUCTIONS

1. In a skillet, heat 2 tbsp. of oil. Add garlic and the rest of the sauce ingredients.
2. Cook until the sauce reduces and ends up being thick.
3. For the filling, warm one tbsp. of oil in another skillet.
4. Add onions and garlic and cook till the onions are caramelized.
5. Add the filling ingredients. Remove from heat and sprinkle Cheddar over the sauce.
6. Take a tortilla and spread a portion of the sauce on it.

7. Add the filling. Roll up the tortilla cautiously. Repeat for each tortilla.
8. Line a baking pan with aluminum foil. Preheat the Air Fryer to 160° C and cook for 15 minutes.
9. Turn the tortillas over in the middle of to cook uniformly.

9. Easy Vegan Air Fryer Brussels Sprouts

INGREDIENTS

- 1-pound Brussels Sprouts
- 2 tsp olive oil
- 1/4 tsp salt
- 1/4 tsp garlic powder

INSTRUCTIONS

1. Prepare Brussels sprouts by cutting off the stem and any dark-colored leaves.
2. Place clean Brussels sprouts in a bowl.
3. Add olive oil, salt, and garlic powder to the bowl. Blend well.
4. Place the Brussels sprouts in the air fryer.
5. Cook at 370° F for 6 minutes, removing the crate to shake part of the way through the cooking time. If needed, return the crate to the air fryer and cook for 2-4 additional minutes.

10. Vegetable Momos

INGREDIENTS

For dough:

- 1 ½ cup all-purpose flour
- ½ tsp. salt or to taste
- 5 tbsp. water

For filling:

- 2 cup carrots, grated
- 2 cup cabbage, grated
- 2 tbsp. oil
- 2 tsp. ginger-garlic paste
- 2 tsp. soy sauce
- 2 tsp. vinegar

INSTRUCTIONS

1. Mix the dough ingredients, cover it with plastic wrap and set aside.
2. Sauté the filling ingredients.
3. Fold the dough and cut it into squares. Drop a spoonful of the filling in the center. Wrap the dough around the filling and press edges together.
4. Preheat the Air Fryer to 200° F and cook for 20 minutes. Serve with chili or ketchup.

11. Cornflakes French toast

INGREDIENTS

- Bread slices (brown or white)
- 1 egg white for every 2 slices
- 1 tsp. sugar for every 2 slices
- Crushed cornflakes

INSTRUCTIONS

1. Cut bread slices in half.
2. In a bowl, whisk the egg whites and sugar.
3. Dip the bread into this blend, then spread them with crushed cornflakes.
4. Preheat the Air Fryer to 180° C and cook for 20 minutes.
5. Flip the toast halfway through to cook uniformly.
6. Serve with chocolate sauce.

12. Smoky Air Fryer Chickpeas

INGREDIENTS

- 1 15 oz can chickpeas
- 1 tsp sunflower oil
- 2 tsp lemon juice and 3/4 tsp smoked paprika
- 1/2 tsp ground cumin
- 1/2 tsp garlic
- 1/4 tsp onion
- 1/2 tsp sea salt

INSTRUCTIONS

1. Set your Air Fryer to 390 ° F.
2. Put the rinsed chickpeas in the bin and fry for 12 minutes.
3. Shake bin once at the halfway point.
4. In a medium bowl, mix the oil, lemon and seasonings.

5. Add the seared chickpeas to the bowl of seasonings.
6. Put the prepared chickpeas back in your air fryer basket and set to 360 ° F. Fry for 2-3 minutes more.

13. Mint galette

INGREDIENTS

- 2 cups mint leaves, finely sliced
- 2 medium potatoes, boiled and mashed
- 1 ½ cup coarsely crushed peanuts
- 3 tsp. ginger, finely chopped
- 1-2 tbsp. fresh coriander leaves
- 2 or 3 green chilies, finely chopped
- 1 ½ tbsp. lemon juice
- Salt and pepper to taste

INSTRUCTIONS

1. Blend the cut mint leaves in with the rest of the ingredients in a bowl.
2. Shape into galettes.
3. Wet the galettes with water. Coat each galette with crushed peanuts.
4. Preheat the Air Fryer to 160 F and cook for 25 minutes.
5. Shake occasionally to cook uniformly. Serve with mint chutney or ketchup.

14. Air Fryer Fruit Crumble

INGREDIENTS

- 1 medium apple, finely diced
- 1/2 cup frozen blueberries or strawberries
- 1 1/4 cup brown rice flour
- 2 tsp sugar
- 1/2 tsp ground cinnamon
- 2 tsp nondairy butter

INSTRUCTIONS

1. Preheat air fryer to 350°F for 5 minutes.
2. Place the apple and solidified berries in an air fryer-safe heating skillet or ramekin.
3. In a bowl, mix part of the flour, sugar, cinnamon, and butter.
4. Spoon the flour combo over the fruit.
5. Bake at 350° F for 15 minutes.

15. Palak galette

INGREDIENTS

- 2 tbsp. garam masala
- 2 cups palak leaves
- 1 ½ cup coarsely crushed peanuts
- 3 tsp. ginger finely chopped
- 1-2 tbsp. fresh coriander leaves
- 2 or 3 green chilies finely chopped
- 1 ½ tbsp. lemon juice
- Salt and pepper to taste

INSTRUCTIONS

1. Blend the ingredients in a bowl.
2. Form this blend into round, flat galettes.
3. Wet the galettes with a small amount of water. Coat each galette with crushed peanuts.
4. Preheat the Air Fryer to 160 F for 5 minutes.
5. Place the galettes in the fry bin and let them cook for an additional 25 minutes.
6. Continue turning them over to cook uniformly.
7. Serve with mint chutney or ketchup.

16. Masala French Fries

INGREDIENTS

- 2- medium sized potatoes

For the marinade:

- 1 tbsp. olive oil
- 1 tsp. mixed herbs
- ½- tsp. red chili flakes
- A pinch of salt
- 1 tbsp. lemon juice

INSTRUCTIONS

1. Cut the potato into long slices.
2. Mix the marinade ingredients and add the potato fingers to it.
3. Preheat the Air Fryer to 300 F and cook for 20 or 25 minutes.
4. Shake the fry basket 2-3 times.

17. Dal- Mint Kebab

INGREDIENTS

- cup chickpeas, cooked
- 1 ½- tsp. of ginger-garlic paste
- 1-2 green chilies
- ¼- tsp. red chili powder
- A pinch of salt
- ½- tsp. roasted cumin powder
- tsp. coriander powder
- 1 ½- tbsp. chopped coriander
- ½- tsp. dried mango powder
- 1 cup dry breadcrumbs
- ¼- tsp. black salt
- 1-2 tbsp. all-purpose flour for coating
- 1-2 tbsp. mint
- 1 onion
- ½- cup milk

INSTRUCTIONS

1. Mix chickpeas with the ground ginger and cut green chilies.
2. Pound this mix until it transforms into a thick paste. Add water as required.
3. Add the onions, mint, breadcrumbs and spices. Mix this well until you get a fragile blend.
4. Form into balls.
5. Pour a small amount of milk onto each kebab to wet it. Roll the kebab in the dry breadcrumbs.
6. Preheat the Air Fryer for 5 minutes at 300 F and cook for 30 minutes.
7. Recommended sides for this dish are mint chutney, tomato ketchup or yogurt chutney.

18. Air Fryer Bow Tie Pasta Chips

INGREDIENTS

- 152g dry whole wheat bow tie pasta
- 15ml olive oil
- 7g nutritional yeast
- 3g Italian Seasoning Blend
- 1/2 tsp salt

INSTRUCTIONS

1. Mix the pasta with olive oil, yeast, Italian flavoring, and salt.

2. Cook at 390° F for 5 minutes. Shake the crate and cook for 3-5 minutes more or until crunchy.

19. Barbeque Corn Sandwich

INGREDIENTS

- 2- slices of white bread
- 1 tbsp. softened butter
- 1 cup sweet corn kernels
- 1 small capsicum
- For Barbeque Sauce:
- ¼- tbsp. Worcestershire sauce
- ½- tsp. olive oil
- ½- flake garlic crushed
- ¼- cup chopped onion
- ¼- tbsp. red chili sauce
- ½- cup water

INSTRUCTIONS

1. Cook the sauce ingredients till it thickens. Add the corn to the sauce and mix.
2. Cook the capsicum and strip the skin off. Cut the capsicum into strips.
3. Preheat the Air Fryer to 300 F and cook for 15 minutes.

20. Honey Chili Potatoes

INGREDIENTS

For potatoes:

- 3 large potatoes
- 2 ½ tsp. ginger-garlic paste
- ¼ tsp. salt
- 1 tsp. red chili sauce
- ¼ tsp. red chili powder/black pepper

For sauce:

- 1 capsicum.
- 2 tbsp. olive oil
- 2 onions, halved
- 1 ½ tbsp. sweet chili sauce
- 1 ½ tsp. ginger garlic paste
- ½ tbsp. red chili sauce.
- 2 tbsp. tomato ketchup
- 2 tsp. soy sauce
- 2 tsp. vinegar

- A pinch of black pepper powder
- 1-2 tsp. red chili flakes

INSTRUCTIONS

1. Make the sauce for the potato fingers and coat the chicken well with it.
2. Preheat the Air Fryer to 250 F and cook for 20 minutes.
3. Add the ingredients to the sauce and cook it with the vegetables till it thickens.
4. Add the fingers to the sauce and cook until the flavors have blended.

21. Burger Cutlet

INGREDIENTS:

- 1 large potatoes, boiled and mashed
- ½ cup breadcrumbs
- A pinch of salt to taste
- ¼ tsp. ginger finely chopped
- 1 green chili finely chopped
- 1 tsp. lemon juice
- 1 tbsp. fresh coriander leaves, finely chopped
- ¼ tsp. red chili powder
- ½ cup of boiled peas
- ¼ tsp. cumin powder
- ¼ tsp. dried mango powder

INSTRUCTIONS

1. Combine the ingredients. Form round cutlets with the mixture.
2. Preheat the Air Fryer to 250 F for 5 minutes and cook for 10-12 minutes.
3. Serve hot with mint chutney.

22. Cheese French Fries

INGREDIENTS

- 2 medium potatoes, peeled and cut

For the marinade:

- 1 tbsp. olive oil
- 1 tsp. mixed herbs
- ½ tsp. red chili flakes
- A pinch of salt to taste
- 1 tbsp. lemon juice

For the garnish:

- 1 cup melted cheddar

INSTRUCTIONS

1. Mix marinade ingredients well.
2. Boil the potatoes for around 5 minutes. Dry the potato pieces on a towel.
3. Coat these potato fingers with the marinade.
4. Preheat the Air Fryer to 300 F and cook for 20 or 25 minutes.
5. Sprinkle the cut coriander leaves on the fries. Add cheese and serve hot.

23. Baked Chickpea Stars

INGREDIENTS

- 1 cup white chickpeas, cooked
- 1 tsp. ginger-garlic paste
- 4 tbsp. chopped coriander leaves
- 2 green chilies finely chopped
- 4 tbsp. thick curd
- Pinches of salt and pepper to taste
- 1 tsp. dry mint
- 4 tbsp. roasted sesame seeds
- 2 small onion finely chopped
- ½ tsp. coriander powder
- ½ tsp. cumin powder
- Use olive oil for greasing purposes

INSTRUCTIONS

1. Pound the chickpeas into a paste.
2. Mix the ginger garlic paste, orions, coriander leaves, coriander powder, cumin powder, salt and pepper.
3. Mix with the crushed chickpeas.
4. Spread this mix over a level surface to about a half-inch thickness.
5. Cut star shapes out of this layer.
6. Make a mix of curd and mint leaves and spread this over the outside of the star-shaped cutlets.
7. Coat all of the sides with sesame seeds.
8. Preheat the Air Fryer to 200 F and cook for 30 minutes.
9. Flip the stars in the holder in order to avoid overcooking one side.
10. Serve with mint chutney or tomato ketchup.

24. Air Fried Spicy Cauliflower Stir-Fry

INGREDIENTS

- 1 head cauliflower
- 3/4 cup onion
- 5 cloves garlic
- 1 1/2 tsp tamari
- 1 tsp rice vinegar
- 1 tsp Sriracha
- 1/2 tsp coconut sugar
- 2 scallions for garnish

INSTRUCTIONS

1. Put cauliflower florets in an air fryer. Preheat to 3500 F.
2. Add the cut onion, mix and cook 10 additional minutes.
3. Add garlic, mix and cook 5 additional minutes.
4. Blend soy sauce, rice vinegar, coconut sugar, Sriracha, salt and pepper together in a bowl.
5. Add the blend to cauliflower and mix. Cook 5 additional minutes.

25. Cheesy Spinach Toasties

INGREDIENTS

- 2 toasted bread slices cut into triangles
- 1 tbsp. butter
- 1 tbsp. all-purpose flour
- 1 small onion finely chopped
- 1-2 flakes garlic finely chopped
- Half a bunch of spinach
- 1 tsp. coarsely crushed green chilies
- 2 tbsp. grated pizza cheese
- 1 cup milk
- 1 tbsp. fresh cream
- Some salt and pepper to taste

INSTRUCTIONS

1. Add onions and garlic to a skillet and sauté in butter until the onions are caramelized.
2. Add flour. Continue stewing for 3 minutes.
3. Add milk and keep blending until you heat it to the point of bubbling.
4. Add green chilies, cream, spinach, and seasoning.
5. Mix the ingredients properly and let it cook until mixture thickens.

6. Toast some bread. Apply the paste to the bread.
7. Sprinkle some ground cheese over the paste.
8. Preheat the Air Fryer to 290 F and cook for 10 minutes.

26. Garlic Toast with Cheese

INGREDIENTS

- French bread

Garlic butter:

- 2- tbsp. softened butter
- 4-5- flakes crushed garlic
- A pinch of salt
- ½- tsp. black pepper powder

Topping:

- ¾- cup grated cheese
- 2 tsp. Oregano seasoning
- Red chili flakes

INSTRUCTIONS

1. Mix Garlic Butter ingredients.
2. On each cut of the French bread, spread a part of this garlic butter.
3. Sprinkle some cheese, oregano and chili flakes on top.
4. Preheat the Air Fryer to 240 F and cook for 10 minutes to toast the bread well.

27. Mixed Vegetable Pancakes

INGREDIENTS

- 2 cups shredded vegetables
- 1 ½ cups almond flour
- 3 eggs
- 2 tsp. dried basil
- 2 tsp. dried parsley
- Salt and Pepper to taste
- 3 tbsp. Butter

INSTRUCTIONS

1. Preheat the air fryer to 250 F.

2. In a little bowl, mix the ingredients until smooth.
3. Cook in oil on both sides of the pancake.
4. Serve with maple syrup.

28. Potato Club Sandwich

INGREDIENTS

- 2 slices of white bread
- 1 tbsp. softened butter
- 1 cup boiled potato
- 1 small capsicum

For Barbeque Sauce:

- ¼ tbsp. Worcestershire sauce
- ½ tsp. olive oil
- ½ flake garlic crushed
- ¼ cup chopped onion
- ¼ tbsp. red chili sauce

INSTRUCTIONS

1. Cut the bread diagonally.
2. Cook the sauce ingredients and until it thickens.
3. Add the potato to the sauce and mix. Cook the capsicum and strip the skin off. Cut the capsicum into strips. Assemble sandwich filling between bread slices.
4. Preheat the air fryer for 5 minutes at 300 F and cook for 15 minutes.

29. Air Fryer Cauliflower Chickpea Tacos

INGREDIENTS

- 4 cups cauliflower florets
- 19 -oz can of chickpeas
- 2 tsp olive oil and 2 tsp taco seasoning
- 8 small tortillas and 2 avocados
- 4 cups cabbage shredded
- coconut yogurt to drizzle

INSTRUCTIONS

1. Preheat air fryer to 390° F
2. In a large bowl, mix the cauliflower and chickpeas with olive oil and taco flavoring.
3. Dump everything into the bin of your air fryer.

4. Cook, shaking sporadically, for 15 minutes
5. Serve in tacos with avocado cuts, cabbage, and coconut yogurt.

30. Cottage Cheese Kebab

INGREDIENTS

- 2 cups cubed cottage cheese
- 3 onions chopped
- 5 green chilies-roughly chopped
- 1 ½ tbsp. ginger paste
- 1 ½ tsp. garlic paste
- 1 ½ tsp. salt
- 3 tsp. lemon juice
- 2 tbsp. coriander powder
- 3 tbsp. chopped capsicum
- 2 tbsp. peanut flour
- 3 eggs

INSTRUCTIONS

1. Coat the cheese cubes with the corn flour. Mix ingredients in a bowl.
2. Make the mix into a smooth paste and coat the cubes with the mix.
3. Beat the eggs in a bowl and add salt
4. Dunk the shapes in the egg mix and leave them in the refrigerator for an hour.
5. Preheat the Air Fryer to 290 F and cook for 25 minutes.
6. Serve the kebabs with mint chutney.

31. Cauliflower Garlic and Tamari Stir-Fry

INGREDIENTS

- 1 head cauliflower
- 3/4 cup onion white
- 5 cloves garlic
- 1 1/2 tsp tamari
- 1 tsp rice vinegar
- 1/2 tsp coconut sugar
- 1 tsp Sriracha
- 2 scallions

INSTRUCTIONS

1. Put cauliflower in an air-fryer. Set the temp to 350. Cook 5 minutes.
2. Add the cut onion, mix and cook 5 additional minutes.

3. Add garlic, mix and cook 5 additional minutes.
4. Blend soy sauce, rice vinegar, coconut sugar, Sriracha, salt, and pepper together in a little bowl.
5. Add the blend to cauliflower and mix.
6. Garnish with cut scallions

32. Cottage Cheese Fingers

INGREDIENTS

- 2 cups cottage cheese fingers
- 2 cup dry breadcrumbs
- 2 tsp. oregano
- 2 tsp. red chili flakes

Marinade:

- 1 ½ tbsp. ginger-garlic paste
- 4 tbsp. lemon juice
- 2 tsp. salt
- 1 tsp. pepper powder
- 1 tsp. red chili powder
- 6 tbsp. corn flour
- 4 eggs

INSTRUCTIONS

1. Blend all of the components for the marinade and soak the cheese fingers.
2. Blend the breadcrumbs, oregano and red chili well and cover the marinated fingers with this mix.
3. Preheat the Air Fryer to 160 and cook for 15 minutes.

33. Roasted Broccoli with Cheese Sauce

INGREDIENTS

- 6- cups broccoli florets
- 10- tsp low-fat evaporated milk
- 1 1/2- oz. queso fresco
- 4 - tsp yellow curry paste
- 6 lower-sodium saltine crackers

INSTRUCTIONS

1. Coat broccoli florets well with cooking oil.
2. Put broccoli florets into fryer basket, and cook at 375°F for 6 to 8 minutes.

3. Blend milk, queso fresco, curry paste, and saltines in a blender; process until smooth, about 45 seconds.
4. Put sauce into a microwaveable bowl.
5. Microwave on high until warm, about 30 seconds
6. Serve cheese sauce with broccoli.

34. Cottage Cheese Croquette

INGREDIENTS

- 2 packets cottage cheese, cubed

1st Marinade:

- 3 tbsp. vinegar or lemon juice
- 2 or 3 tsp. paprika
- 1 tsp. black pepper
- 1 tsp. salt
- 3 tsp. ginger-garlic paste

2nd Marinade:

- 1 cup yogurt
- 4 tsp. tandoori masala
- 2 tbsp. dry fenugreek leaves
- 1 tsp. black salt
- 1 tsp. chat masala
- 1 tsp. garam masala powder
- 1 tsp. red chili powder
- 1 tsp. salt
- 3 drops of red color

INSTRUCTIONS

1. Make the 1st marinade and drench the cubed curds in it for 4 hours.
2. Make the 2nd marinade and sprinkle the curds in it to let the flavors blend.
3. Preheat the Air Fryer to 160 F and cook for 15 minutes.
4. Serve with mint chutney.

35. Onion Galette

INGREDIENTS

- 2 tbsp. garam masala
- 2 medium onions (Cut long)
- 1 ½ cup coarsely crushed peanuts
- 3 tsp. ginger finely chopped

- 1-2 tbsp. fresh coriander leaves
- 2 or 3 green chilies finely chopped
- 1 ½ tbsp. lemon juice
- Salt and pepper to taste

INSTRUCTIONS

1. Blend the ingredients in a bowl.
2. Shape this blend into round and level galettes.
3. Wet the galettes marginally with water. Coat each galette with crushed peanuts.
4. Preheat the Air Fryer to 160 and cook for 25 minutes.
5. Serve either with mint chutney or ketchup.

36. Cauliflower galette

INGREDIENTS

- 2 tbsp. garam masala
- 2 cups cauliflower
- 1 ½ cup coarsely crushed peanuts
- 3 tsp. ginger finely chopped
- 1-2 tbsp. fresh coriander leaves
- 2 or 3 green chilies finely chopped
- 1 ½ tbsp. lemon juice
- Salt and pepper to taste

INSTRUCTIONS

1. Blend the ingredients in a bowl.
2. Form this blend into round, flat galettes.
3. Wet the galettes with a small amount of water. Coat each galette with crushed peanuts.
4. Preheat the Air Fryer to 160 F for 5 minutes.
5. Place the galettes in the fry bin and let them cook for an additional 25 minutes.
6. Continue turning them over to cook uniformly.
7. Serve with mint chutney or ketchup.

37. Cabbage Galette

INGREDIENTS

- 2 tbsp. garam masala
- 2 cups cabbage
- 1 ½ cup coarsely crushed peanuts
- 3 tsp. ginger finely chopped
- 1-2 tbsp. fresh coriander leaves

- 2 or 3 green chilies finely chopped
- 1 ½ tbsp. lemon juice
- Salt and pepper to taste

1. Blend the ingredients in a bowl.
2. Form this blend into round and level galettes.
3. Wet the galettes marginally with water. Coat each galette with crushed peanuts.
4. Preheat the Air Fryer to 160 and cook for 25 minutes. Continue turning them over to cook uniformly.
5. Serve either with mint chutney or ketchup.

38. Cottage Cheese Galette

INGREDIENTS

- 2 tbsp. garam masala
- 2 cups grated cottage cheese
- 1 ½ cup coarsely crushed peanuts
- 3 tsp. ginger finely chopped
- 1-2 tbsp. fresh coriander leaves
- 2 or 3 green chilies finely chopped
- 1 ½ tbsp. lemon juice
- Salt and pepper to taste

INSTRUCTIONS

1. Blend the ingredients in a bow .
2. Form this blend into round and level galettes.
3. Wet the galettes somewhat with water. Coat each galette with crushed peanuts.
4. Preheat the Air Fryer to 160 and cook for 25 minutes. Continue turning them over to cook uniformly.
5. Serve either with mint chutney or ketchup.

39. Gourd Galette

INGREDIENTS

- 2 tbsp. garam masala
- 2 cups sliced gourd
- 1 ½ cup coarsely crushed peanuts
- 3 tsp. ginger finely chopped
- 1-2 tbsp. fresh coriander leaves
- 2 or 3 green chilies finely chopped
- 1 ½ tbsp. lemon juice
- Salt and pepper to taste

INSTRUCTIONS

1. Blend the ingredients in a bowl.

2. Form this blend into round and level galettes.
3. Wet the galettes somewhat with water. Coat each galette with crushed peanuts.
4. Preheat the Air Fryer to 160 and cook for 25 minutes. Continue turning them over to cook uniformly.
5. Serve either with mint chutney or ketchup.

40. Cottage Cheese Club Sandwich

INGREDIENTS

- 2 slices of white bread
- 1 tbsp. softened butter
- 1 cup sliced cottage cheese
- 1 small capsicum
- For Barbeque Sauce:
- ¼ tbsp. Worcestershire sauce
- ½ tsp. olive oil
- ½ flake garlic crushed
- ¼ cup chopped onion
- ¼ tbsp. red chili sauce

INSTRUCTIONS

1. Cook the sauce ingredients and until it thickens.
2. Add the cheese to the sauce and mix.
3. Cook the capsicum and strip the skin off. Cut the capsicum into strips.
4. Preheat the Air Fryer for 5 minutes at 300 F and cook for 15 minutes.
5. Serve the sandwiches with tomato ketchup or mint chutney.

41. Cottage Cheese Patties

INGREDIENTS

- 1 cup grated cottage cheese
- A pinch of salt to taste
- ¼ tsp. ginger finely chopped
- 1 green chili finely chopped
- 1 tsp. lemon juice
- 1 tbsp. fresh coriander leaves
- ¼ tsp. red chili powder
- ¼ tsp. cumin powder

INSTRUCTIONS

1. Combine the ingredients. Make round patties.

2. Preheat the Air Fryer to 250 F and cook for 10 or 12 minutes, flipping halfway through.
3. Serve warm with mint chutney.

42. Pineapple Kebab

INGREDIENTS

- 2 cups cubed pineapples
- 3 onions chopped
- 5 green chilies-roughly chopped
- 1 ½ tbsp. ginger paste
- 1 ½ tsp. garlic paste
- 1 ½ tsp. salt
- 3 tsp. lemon juice
- 2 tsp. garam masala
- 4 tbsp. chopped coriander
- 3 tbsp. cream
- 3 tbsp. chopped capsicum
- 3 eggs
- 2 ½ tbsp. white sesame seeds

INSTRUCTIONS

1. Pound the ingredients except for the pineapple and egg to create a smooth paste.
2. Coat the pineapples in the paste.
3. Beat the eggs and add salt.
4. Dip the pineapples in the egg blend and then coat with sesame seeds. Place on skewers.
5. Preheat the Air Fryer to 160 F and cook for 25 minutes.
6. Turn the sticks over in the middle of the cooking procedure to cook uniformly.

43. Broccoli Tikka

INGREDIENTS

- 2 cups broccoli florets
- 3 onions chopped
- 5 green chilies-roughly chopped
- 1 ½ tbsp. ginger paste
- 1 ½ tsp. garlic paste
- 1 ½ tsp. salt
- 3 tsp. lemon juice
- 2 tsp. garam masala
- 3 eggs
- 2 ½ tbsp. white sesame seeds

INSTRUCTIONS

1. Crush the ingredients aside from the broccoli and egg and make a smooth paste.
2. Coat the broccoli in the paste. Beat the eggs and add salt.
3. Dip the broccoli in the egg blend and then coat with sesame seeds. Place on skewers.
4. Preheat the Air Fryer to 160 F and cook for 25 minutes.
5. Turn the sticks over in the middle of the cooking procedure to cook uniformly.

44. Cabbage Fritters

INGREDIENTS

- 10 leaves cabbage
- 3 onions chopped
- 5 green chilies-roughly chopped
- 1 ½ tbsp. ginger paste
- 1 ½ tsp. garlic paste
- 1 ½ tsp. salt
- 3 tsp. lemon juice
- 2 tsp. garam masala
- 3 eggs
- 2 ½ tbsp. white sesame seeds

INSTRUCTIONS

1. Crush the ingredients aside from the cabbage and egg and make a smooth paste.
2. Coat the cabbage in the paste. Beat the eggs and add salt.
3. Dip the cabbage in the egg blend and then coat with sesame seeds. Place on skewers.
4. Preheat the Air Fryer to 160 F and cook for 25 minutes.
5. Turn the sticks over in the middle of the cooking procedure to cook uniformly.

45. Cottage Cheese Gnocchi

INGREDIENTS

For dough:

- 1 ½ cup all-purpose flour
- ½ tsp. salt
- 5 tbsp. water

For filling:

- 2 cups grated cottage cheese
- 2 tbsp. oil
- 2 tsp. ginger-garlic paste
- 2 tsp. soy sauce
- 2 tsp. vinegar

INSTRUCTIONS

1. Make the dough, spread it with saran wrap and set aside.
2. Combine the filling ingredients.
3. Roll the dough and place the filling in the middle.
4. Presently, wrap the dough to cover the filling and squeeze the edges together.
5. Preheat the Air Fryer to 200° F and cook for 20 minutes.

46. Cauliflower Gnocchi

INGREDIENTS

For dough:

- 1 ½ cup all-purpose flour
- ½ tsp. salt
- 5 tbsp. water

For filling:

- 2 cups grated cauliflower
- 2 tbsp. oil
- 2 tsp. ginger-garlic paste
- 2 tsp. soy sauce
- 2 tsp. vinegar

INSTRUCTIONS

1. 1.Make the dough, spread it with saran wrap and set aside.
2. 2.Combine the filling ingredients.
3. 3.Roll the dough and place the filling n the middle.
4. Presently, wrap the dough to cover the filling and squeeze the edges together.
5. Preheat the Air Fryer to 200° F and cook for 20 minutes.

47. Air Fryer Roasted Broccoli and Cauliflower

INGREDIENTS

- 3 cups broccoli florets
- 3 cups cauliflower florets
- 2 tsp olive oil
- ¼ tsp paprika
- ½ tsp garlic powder
- ⅛ tsp black pepper
- ¼ tsp sea salt

INSTRUCTIONS

1. Preheat an air fryer to 400 F.
2. Put broccoli florets in a large microwave-safe bowl. Cook on high for 3 minutes.
3. Add cauliflower, olive oil, garlic powder, ocean salt, paprika, and pepper to the bowl with the broccoli.
4. Place in the air fryer basket. Cook for 12 minutes.

48. Broccoli Momos

INGREDIENTS

For dough:

- 1 ½ cup all-purpose flour
- ½ tsp. salt
- 5 tbsp. water

For filling:

- 2 cups grated broccoli
- 2 tbsp. oil
- 2 tsp. ginger-garlic paste
- 2 tsp. soy sauce
- 2 tsp. vinegar

INSTRUCTIONS

1. Make the dough, spread it with saran wrap and set aside.
2. Combine the filling ingredients.
3. Roll the dough and place the filling in the middle.
4. Presently, wrap the dough to cover the filling and squeeze the edges together.
5. Preheat the Air Fryer to 200° F and cook for 20 minutes.

49. Cauliflower Momos

INGREDIENTS

For dough:

- 1 ½ cup all-purpose flour
- ½ tsp. salt
- 5 tbsp. water

For filling:

- 2 cups grated cauliflower
- 2 tbsp. oil
- 2 tsp. ginger-garlic paste
- 2 tsp. soy sauce
- 2 tsp. vinegar

INSTRUCTIONS

1. Make the dough, spread it with saran wrap and set aside.
2. Combine the filling ingredients.
3. Roll the dough and place the filling in the middle.
4. Presently, wrap the dough to cover the filling and squeeze the edges together.
5. Preheat the Air Fryer to 200° F and cook for 20 minutes.

50. Aloo Patties

INGREDIENTS

- 1 cup mashed potato
- A pinch of salt to taste
- ¼ tsp. ginger finely chopped
- 1 green chili finely chopped
- 1 tsp. lemon juice
- 1 tbsp. fresh coriander leaves
- ¼ tsp. red chili powder
- ¼ tsp. cumin powder

INSTRUCTIONS

1. Combine the ingredients and make round patties.
2. Preheat the Air Fryer to 250 F and cook for 10 or 12 minutes, flipping halfway through.
3. Serve warm with mint chutney.

51. Mixed Vegetable Patties

INGREDIENTS:

- 1 cup grated mixed vegetables
- A pinch of salt to taste
- ¼ tsp. ginger finely chopped
- 1 green chili finely chopped
- 1 tsp. lemon juice
- 1 tbsp. fresh coriander leaves
- ¼ tsp. red chili powder
- ¼ tsp. cumin powder

INSTRUCTIONS

1. Combine the ingredients and make round patties.
2. Preheat the Air Fryer to 250 F and cook for 10 or 12 minutes, flipping halfway through.
3. Serve warm with mint chutney

52. Cottage Cheese Momos

INGREDIENTS

For dough:

- 1 ½ cup all-purpose flour
- ½ tsp. salt
- 5 tbsp. water

For filling:

- 2 cups crumbled cottage cheese
- 2 tbsp. oil
- 2 tsp. ginger-garlic paste
- 2 tsp. soy sauce
- 2 tsp. vinegar

INSTRUCTIONS

1. Make the dough, spread it with saran wrap and set aside.
2. Combine the filling ingredients.
3. Roll the dough and place the filling in the middle.
4. Wrap the dough to cover the filling and squeeze the edges together.
5. Preheat the Air Fryer to 200° F and cook for 20 minutes.

53. Mushroom Galette

INGREDIENTS

- 2 tbsp. garam masala
- 2 cups sliced mushrooms
- ½ cup coarsely crushed peanuts
- 3 tsp. ginger finely chopped
- 1-2 tbsp. fresh coriander leaves
- 2 or 3 green chilies finely chopped
- 1 ½ tbsp. lemon juice
- Salt and pepper to taste

INSTRUCTIONS

1. Blend the ingredients in a bowl.
2. Form this blend into round and leve galettes.
3. Wet the galettes somewhat with water. Coat each galette with crushed peanuts.
4. Preheat the Air Fryer to 160 and cook for 25 minutes.
5. Continue turning them over to cook uniformly.
6. Serve either with mint chutney or ketchup.

54. Zucchini Samosa

INGREDIENTS

- 2 tbsp. unsalted butter
- 1 ½ cup all-purpose flour
- A pinch of salt
- water

For filling:

- 3 medium zucchinis
- ¼ cup boiled peas
- 1 tsp. powdered ginger
- 1 or 2 green chilies
- ½ tsp. cumin
- 1 tsp. coarsely crushed coriander
- 1 dry red chili
- A small amount of salt
- ½ tsp. dried mango powder
- ½ tsp. red chili powder.
- 1-2 tbsp. coriander.

INSTRUCTIONS

1. Create the dough with the first 4 ingredients. Set aside.

2. Cook the filling ingredients in skillet and blend them well to make a thick paste.
3. Form the paste into balls. Cut them in half and insert the filling.
4. Preheat the Air Fryer to 300 F. Place the samosas in the fry receptacle.
5. Cook for 20 to 25 minutes. Around the midpoint, turn the samosas over for uniform cooking.
6. Serve hot with tamarind or mint chutney.

55. Vegetable Skewer

INGREDIENTS

- 2 cups mixed vegetables
- 3 onions chopped
- 5 green chilies
- 1 ½ tbsp. ginger paste
- 1 ½ tsp. garlic paste
- 1 ½ tsp. salt
- 3 tbsp. cream
- 3 eggs
- 2 ½ tbsp. white sesame seeds

INSTRUCTIONS

1. 1.Crush the ingredients aside from the mixed vegetables and egg and make a smooth paste.
2. Coat with the paste. Beat the eggs and add salt.
3. Dip the cabbage in the egg blend and then coat with sesame seeds. Place on skewers.
4. Preheat the Air Fryer to 160 F and cook for 25 minutes.
5. Turn the sticks over in the middle of the cooking procedure to cook uniformly.

56. Black Gram Galette

INGREDIENTS

- 2 cup black gram
- 2 medium potatoes boiled and mashed
- 1 ½ cup coarsely crushed peanuts
- 3 tsp. ginger finely chopped
- 1-2 tbsp. fresh coriander leaves
- 2 or 3 green chilies finely chopped
- 1 ½ tbsp. lemon juice
- Salt and pepper to taste

INSTRUCTIONS

1. Blend the ingredients in a bowl.
2. Form this blend into round and level galettes.
3. Wet the galettes somewhat with water. Coat each galette with crushed peanuts.
4. Preheat the Air Fryer to 160 and cook for 25 minutes. Continue turning them over to cook uniformly.
5. Serve either with mint chutney or ketchup.

57. Stuffed Eggplant Baskets

INGREDIENTS

For baskets:

- 6 eggplants
- ½ tsp. salt
- ½ tsp. pepper powder

For filling:

- 1 medium onion finely chopped
- 1 green chili finely chopped
- 1 ½ tbsp. chopped coriander leaves
- 1 tsp. fenugreek
- 1 tsp. dried mango powder
- 1 tsp. cumin powder
- Salt and pepper to taste
- For topping:
- 3 tbsp. grated cheese
- 1 tsp. red chili flakes
- ½ tsp. oregano
- ½ tsp. basil
- ½ tsp. parsley

INSTRUCTIONS

1. Mix filling ingredients in a bowl.
2. Remove the stem of the eggplant and slice. Season with salt and pepper.
3. Fill the eggplant with the filling, leaving a little space at the top.
4. Sprinkle cheese and topping spices on top.
5. Preheat the Air Fryer to 140 F and cook for 20 minutes, flipping halfway through.

58. Mushroom Pasta

INGREDIENTS

- 1 cup pasta, cooked
- 1 ½ tbsp. olive oil
- A pinch of salt

For tossing pasta:

- 1 ½ tbsp. olive oil
- Salt and pepper to taste
- ½ tsp. oregano
- ½ tsp. basil

For sauce:

- 2 tbsp. olive oil
- 2 cups sliced mushroom
- 2 tbsp. all-purpose flour
- 2 cups of milk
- 1 tsp. dried oregano
- ½ tsp. dried basil
- ½ tsp. dried parsley
- Salt and pepper to taste

INSTRUCTIONS

1. For the sauce, add the ingredients to a container and boil.
2. Mix the sauce and keep on stewing to thicken it.
3. Add the pasta to the sauce and move this into a glass bowl embellished with cheese.
4. Preheat the Air Fryer to 160 C and cook for 10 minutes.

59. Mushroom Samosa

INGREDIENTS

For wrappers:

- 1 cup all-purpose flour
- 2 tbsp. unsalted butter
- A pinch of salt

For filling:

- 3 cups whole mushrooms
- 2 onions sliced
- 2 capsicum sliced
- 2 carrots sliced
- 2 cabbage sliced
- 2 tbsp. soy sauce
- 2 tsp. vinegar
- 2 tbsp. green chilies finely chopped
- 2 tbsp. ginger-garlic paste
- Some salt and pepper to taste

INSTRUCTIONS

1. Create the dough with the first 4 ingredients. Set aside.
2. Cook the filling ingredients in skillet and blend them well to make a thick paste.
3. Form the paste into balls. Cut them in half and insert the filling.
4. Preheat the Air Fryer to 300 F. Place the samosas in the fry receptacle.
5. Cook for 20 to 25 minutes. Around the midpoint, turn the samosas over for uniform cooking.
6. Serve hot with tamarind or mint chutney

60. Cottage Cheese and Mushroom Burritos

INGREDIENTS

Refried beans:

- ½ cup red kidney beans
- ½ small onion chopped
- 1 tbsp. olive oil
- 2 tbsp. tomato puree
- ¼ tsp. red chili powder
- 1 tsp. of salt to taste
- 4-5 flour tortillas
- Vegetable Filling:
- ½ cup mushrooms thinly sliced
- 1 cup cottage cheese
- A pinch of salt to taste
- ½ tsp. red chili flakes
- 1 tsp. freshly ground peppercorns
- ½ cup pickled Jalapeño s

Salad:

- 1-2 lettuce leaves shredded.
- 1 or 2 spring onions
- Take one tomato.
- 1 green chili chopped.
- 1 cup of Cheddar grated.

To serve:

- 1 cup boiled rice
- A few flour tortillas

INSTRUCTIONS

1. Cook the beans with the onion and garlic and mash them.
2. For the filling, sauté the ingredients in a pan.
3. Toss the salad ingredients together.
4. Lay the tortilla on a flat surface and place a layer of sauce and filling inside.
5. Wrap the tortilla to create a burrito.
6. Preheat the Air Fryer to 200 F. Open the fry case and place the burritos inside.
7. Cook for 15 minutes. Flip the burritos halfway through.

61. French Bean Toast

INGREDIENTS

- Bread slices (brown or white)
- 1 egg white for every 2 slices
- 1 tsp. sugar for every 2 slices
- Crushed cornflakes
- 2 cups baked beans

INSTRUCTIONS

1. In a bowl, whisk the egg whites and sugar.
2. Plunge the bread triangles into this blend and then cover them with crushed cornflakes.
3. Preheat the Air Fryer to 180° C and cook for 20 minutes. Top with prepared beans and serve.

62. Mushroom Pops

INGREDIENTS

- 1 cup whole mushrooms
- 1 ½ tsp. garlic paste
- Salt and pepper to taste
- 1 tsp. dry oregano
- 1 tsp. dry basil
- 1 tsp. lemon juice
- 1 tsp. red chili flakes

INSTRUCTIONS

1. Mix the ingredients except mushrooms in a bowl.
2. Dunk the mushrooms in the above blend and set them aside.
3. Preheat the Air Fryer to 180° C and cook for 20 minutes.

63. Potato Pancakes

INGREDIENTS

- 2 tbsp. garam masala
- 2 cups sliced potato
- 3 tsp. ginger finely chopped
- 1-2 tbsp. fresh coriander leaves
- 2 or 3 green chilies finely chopped
- 1 ½ tbsp. lemon juice
- Salt and pepper to taste

INSTRUCTIONS

1. Blend the ingredients in a bowl and add water to it.
2. Preheat the Air Fryer to 160 F and cook for 25 minutes.
3. Continue turning them over to cook uniformly.
4. Serve either with mint chutney or ketchup.

64. Cottage Cheese Pancakes

INGREDIENTS

- 2 tbsp. garam masala
- 2 cups sliced cottage cheese
- 3 tsp. ginger finely chopped
- 1-2 tbsp. fresh coriander leaves
- 2 or 3 green chilies finely chopped
- 1 ½ tbsp. lemon juice
- Salt and pepper to taste

INSTRUCTIONS

1. Blend the ingredients in a bowl and add water to it.
2. Preheat the Air Fryer to 160 F and cook for 25 minutes.
3. Continue turning them over to cook uniformly.
4. Serve either with mint chutney or ketchup.

65. Fenugreek Galette

INGREDIENTS

- 2 cups fenugreek
- 2 medium potatoes, boiled and mashed
- 3 tsp. ginger finely chopped
- 1-2 tbsp. fresh coriander leaves
- 2 or 3 green chilies finely chopped
- 1 ½ tbsp. lemon juice
- Salt and pepper to taste

INSTRUCTIONS

1. Blend the ingredients in a bowl.
2. Form this blend into round and level galettes.
3. Wet the galettes somewhat with water.
4. Preheat the Air Fryer to 160 F and cook for 25 minutes.
5. Continue turning them over to cook uniformly.
6. Serve either with mint chutney or ketchup.

66. Potato Wedges

INGREDIENTS

- 2 medium sized potatoes

For the marinade:

- 1 tbsp. olive oil
- 1 tsp. mixed herbs
- ½ tsp. red chili flakes
- A pinch of salt to taste
- 1 tbsp. lemon juice

INSTRUCTIONS

1. Cut the potatoes into wedges.
2. Blend marinade ingredients and pour over potato fingers, ensuring that they are covered well.
3. Preheat the Air Fryer to 300 F and cook for 20 or 25 minutes. Toss the fries 2-3 times.

67. Potato Kebab

INGREDIENTS

- 2 cups sliced potato
- 1 1/2 tsp. of ginger-garlic paste
- 1-2 green chilies, chopped finely
- ¼ tsp. red chili powder
- A pinch of salt
- ½ tsp. cumin powder
- 2 tsp. coriander powder
- 1 ½ tbsp. chopped fresh coriander
- ½ tsp. dried mango powder
- 1 cup dry breadcrumbs
- ¼ tsp. black salt
- 1-2 tbsp. flour
- 1-2 tbsp. mint, finely chopped)
- 1 onion, finely chopped
- ½ cup milk

INSTRUCTIONS

1. Mix the potato slices with the ground ginger and cut green chilies.
2. Pound this blend until it turns into a thick paste. Add water if required.
3. Add the onions, mint, breadcrumbs and spices. Blend this well until you get a soft mixture.
4. Form round kebabs with the dough.
5. Pour a small amount of milk onto each kebab to wet it.
6. Roll the kebab in the dry breadcrumbs.
7. Preheat the Air Fryer for 5 minutes at 300 F and cook for 30 minutes.
8. Recommended sides for this dish are mint chutney, tomato ketchup or yogurt chutney.

68. Cabbage Pancakes

INGREDIENTS

- 2 tbsp. garam masala
- 2 cups halved cabbage leaves
- 3 tsp. ginger finely chopped
- 1-2 tbsp. fresh coriander leaves
- 2 or 3 green chilies finely chopped
- 1 ½ tbsp. lemon juice
- Salt and pepper to taste

INSTRUCTIONS

1. Blend the ingredients in a bowl and add water to it.
2. Preheat the Air Fryer to 160 F and cook for 25 minutes.
3. Continue turning them over to cook uniformly.
4. Serve either with mint chutney or ketchup.

69. Bitter Gourd Pancakes

INGREDIENTS

- 2 tbsp. garam masala
- 2 cups sliced bitter gourd
- 3 tsp. ginger finely chopped
- 1-2 tbsp. fresh coriander leaves
- 2 or 3 green chilies finely chopped
- 1 ½ tbsp. lemon juice
- Salt and pepper to taste

INSTRUCTIONS

1. Blend the ingredients in a bowl and add water to it.
2. Preheat the Air Fryer to 160 F and cook for 25 minutes.
3. Continue turning them over to cook uniformly.
4. Serve either with mint chutney or ketchup.

70. Pumpkin Galette

INGREDIENTS

- 2 tbsp. garam masala
- 1 cup sliced pumpkin
- 3 tsp. ginger finely chopped
- 1-2 tbsp. fresh coriander leaves
- 2 or 3 green chilies finely chopped
- 1 ½ tbsp. lemon juice
- Salt and pepper to taste

INSTRUCTIONS

1. Blend the ingredients in a bowl.
2. Form this blend into round, flat galettes.
3. Wet the galettes with a small amount of water. Coat each galette with crushed peanuts.
4. Preheat the Air Fryer to 160 F for 5 minutes.
5. Place the galettes in the fry bin and let them cook for an additional 25 minutes.
6. Continue turning them over to cook uniformly.
7. Serve with mint chutney or ketchup.

71. Masala Potato Wedges

INGREDIENTS

- 2 medium sized potatoes (Cut into wedges)

For the marinade:

- 1 tbsp. olive oil
- 1 tsp. garam masala
- 1 tsp. mixed herbs
- ½ tsp. red chili flakes
- A pinch of salt to taste
- 1 tbsp. lemon juice

INSTRUCTIONS

1. Cut the potatoes into wedges.
2. Blend marinade ingredients and pour over potato fingers, ensuring that they are covered well.
3. Preheat the Air Fryer to 300 F and cook for 20 or 25 minutes. Toss the fries 2-3 times.

72. Cheesy Potato Wedges

INGREDIENTS

- 2 medium sized potatoes (Cut into wedges)
- for the marinade:
- 1 tbsp. olive oil
- 1 tsp. mixed herbs
- ½ tsp. red chili flakes
- A pinch of salt to taste
- 1 tbsp. lemon juice
- 1 cup molten cheese

INSTRUCTIONS

1. Cut the potatoes into wedges.
2. Blend marinade ingredients and pour over potato fingers, ensuring that they are covered well.
3. Preheat the Air Fryer to 300 F and cook for 20 or 25 minutes.
4. Toss the fries 2-3 times.

73. Asparagus Pancakes

INGREDIENTS

- 2 tbsp. garam masala
- 2 cups sliced asparagus
- 3 tsp. ginger finely chopped
- 1-2 tbsp. fresh coriander leaves
- 2 or 3 green chilies finely chopped
- 1 ½ tbsp. lemon juice
- Salt and pepper to taste

INSTRUCTIONS

1. Blend the ingredients in a bowl and add water to it.
2. Preheat the Air Fryer to 160 F and cook for 25 minutes.
3. Continue turning them over to cook uniformly.
4. Serve either with mint chutney or ketchup.

74. Mushroom Wonton

INGREDIENTS

For dough:

- 1 ½ cup all-purpose flour
- ½ tsp. salt or to taste
- 5 tbsp. water

For filling:

- 2 cups cubed mushroom
- 2 tbsp. oil
- 2 tsp. ginger-garlic paste
- 2 tsp. soy sauce
- 2 tsp. vinegar

INSTRUCTIONS

1. Mix the dough ingredients, cover with cling wrap and set aside.
2. Cook the filling ingredients.
3. Roll the dough and place the filling in the middle.
4. Wrap the dough to cover the filling and squeeze the edges together.
5. Preheat the Air Fryer to 200° F and cook for 20 minutes.

75. Mushroom Patties

INGREDIENTS

- 1 cup minced mushroom
- A pinch of salt to taste
- ¼ tsp. ginger finely chopped
- 1 green chili finely chopped
- 1 tsp. lemon juice
- 1 tbsp. fresh coriander leaves
- ¼ tsp. red chili powder
- ¼ tsp. cumin powder

INSTRUCTIONS

1. Combine the ingredients. Make round patties.
2. Preheat the Air Fryer to 250 F and cook for 10 or 12 minutes, flipping halfway through.
3. Serve warm with mint chutney.

76. Cheese and Mushroom Kebab

INGREDIENTS

- 2 cups sliced mushrooms
- 1-2 green chilies chopped finely
- ¼ tsp. red chili powder
- A pinch of salt to taste
- ½ tsp. dried mango powder
- ¼ tsp. black salt
- 1-2 tbsp. all-purpose flour for coating purposes
- 1-2 tbsp. mint
- 1 cup molten cheese
- 1 onion that has been finely chopped
- ½ cup milk

INSTRUCTIONS

1. Mix the mushroom slices with the ground ginger and cut green chilies.
2. Pound this blend until it turns into a thick paste.
3. Add water if required. Add the onions, mint, breadcrumbs and spices.
4. Blend this well until you get a soft mixture.
5. Form round kebabs with the dough.
6. Pour a small amount of milk onto each kebab to wet it.
7. Roll the kebab in the dry breadcrumbs.
8. Preheat the Air Fryer for 5 minutes at 300 F and cook for 30 minutes.
9. Recommended sides for this dish are mint chutney, tomato ketchup or yogurt chutney.

77. Mushroom Club Sandwich

INGREDIENTS

- 2 slices of white bread
- 1 tbsp. softened butter
- 1 cup minced mushroom
- 1 small capsicum

For Barbeque Sauce:

- ¼ tbsp. Worcestershire sauce
- ½ tsp. olive oil
- ½ flake garlic crushed
- ¼ cup chopped onion
- ¼ tbsp. red chili sauce
- ½ cup water

INSTRUCTIONS

1. Cook the sauce ingredients and until it thickens.
2. Add the cheese to the sauce and mix.
3. Cook the capsicum and strip the skin off. Cut the capsicum into strips.
4. Preheat the Air Fryer for 5 minutes at 300 F and cook for 15 minutes.
5. Spread on the pieces of bread and serve sandwiches with tomato ketchup or mint chutney.

78. Asparagus Galette

INGREDIENTS

- 2 cups minced asparagus
- 3 tsp. ginger finely chopped
- 1-2 tbsp. fresh coriander leaves
- 2 or 3 green chilies finely chopped
- 1 ½ tbsp. lemon juice
- Salt and pepper to taste

INSTRUCTIONS

1. Blend the ingredients in a bowl.
2. Shape this blend into round and level galettes.
3. Wet the galettes marginally with water.
4. Preheat the Air Fryer to 160 F and cook for 25 minutes.
5. Continue turning them over to cook uniformly.
6. Serve either with mint chutney or ketchup.

79. Asparagus Kebab

INGREDIENTS

- 2 cups sliced asparagus
- 3 onions chopped
- 5 green chilies-roughly chopped

- 1 ½ tbsp. ginger paste
- 1 ½ tsp. garlic paste
- 1 ½ tsp. salt
- 3 tsp. lemon juice
- 2 tsp. garam masala
- 3 eggs
- 2 ½ tbsp. white sesame seeds

INSTRUCTIONS

1. Mix the asparagus with the ground ginger and cut green chilies.
2. Pound this blend until it turns into a thick paste.
3. Add water if required. Add the onions, mint, breadcrumbs and spices.
4. Blend this well until you get a soft mixture.
5. Form round kebabs with the dough.
6. Pour a small amount of milk onto each kebab to wet it.
7. Roll the kebab in the dry breadcrumbs.
8. Preheat the Air Fryer for 5 minutes at 300 F and cook for 30 minutes.
9. Recommended sides for this dish are mint chutney, tomato ketchup or yogurt chutney.

80. Green Chili Pancakes

INGREDIENTS

- 2 tbsp. garam masala
- 10–12 green chilies
- 3 tsp. ginger finely chopped
- 1-2 tbsp. fresh coriander leaves
- 2 or 3 green chilies finely chopped
- 1 ½ tbsp. lemon juice
- Salt and pepper to taste

INSTRUCTIONS

1. Blend the ingredients in a bowl and add water to it.
2. Preheat the Air Fryer to 160 F and cook for 25 minutes.
3. Continue turning them over to cook uniformly.
4. Serve either with mint chutney or ketchup.

81. Cottage Cheese Samosa

INGREDIENTS

- 2 tbsp. unsalted butter
- 1 ½ cup all-purpose flour
- A pinch of salt to taste
- Water

For filling:

- 2 cups mashed cottage cheese
- ¼ cup boiled peas
- 1 tsp. powdered ginger
- 1 or 2 green chilies
- ½ tsp. cumin
- 1 tsp. coarsely crushed coriander
- 1 dry red chili
- A small amount of salt
- ½ tsp. dried mango powder
- ½ tsp. red chili powder
- 1-2 tbsp. coriander

INSTRUCTIONS

1. Create the dough with the first 4 ingredients. Set aside.
2. Cook the filling ingredients in skillet and blend them well to make a thick paste.
3. Form the paste into balls. Cut them in half and insert the filling.
4. Preheat the Air Fryer to 300 F. Place the samosas in the fry receptacle.
5. Cook for 20 to 25 minutes. Around the midpoint, turn the samosas over for uniform cooking.
6. Serve hot with tamarind or mint chutney

82. Taro Gnocchi

INGREDIENTS

For dough:

- 1 ½ cup all-purpose flour
- ½ tsp. salt
- 5 tbsp. water

For filling:

- 2 cups minced taro
- 2 tbsp. oil

- 2 tsp. ginger-garlic paste
- 2 tsp. soy sauce
- 2 tsp. vinegar

INSTRUCTIONS

1. 1.Make the dough, spread it with saran wrap and set aside.
2. 2.Combine the filling ingredients.
3. 3.Roll the dough and place the filling in the middle.
4. Presently, wrap the dough to cover the filling and squeeze the edges together.
5. 4.Preheat the Air Fryer to 200° F and cook for 20 minutes.

83. Okra Kebab

INGREDIENTS

- 2 cups sliced okra
- 3 onions chopped
- 5 green chilies-roughly chopped
- 1 ½ tbsp. ginger paste
- 1 ½ tsp. garlic paste
- 1 ½ tsp. salt
- 3 tsp. lemon juice
- 2 tsp. garam masala
- 4 tbsp. chopped coriander
- 3 tbsp. cream
- 3 tbsp. chopped capsicum
- 3 eggs
- 2 ½ tbsp. white sesame seeds

INSTRUCTIONS

1. Mix the okra with the ground ginger and cut green chilies.
2. Pound this blend until it turns into a thick paste. Add water if required.
3. Add the onions, mint, breadcrumbs and spices. Blend this well until you get a soft mixture.
4. Form round kebabs with the dough.
5. Pour a small amount of milk onto each kebab to wet it.
6. Roll the kebab in the dry breadcrumbs.
7. Preheat the Air Fryer for 5 minutes at 300 F and cook for 30 minutes.
8. Recommended sides for this dish are mint chutney, tomato ketchup or yogurt chutney.

84. Okra Pancakes

INGREDIENTS

- 2 tbsp. garam masala
- 2 cups sliced okra
- 3 tsp. ginger finely chopped
- 1-2 tbsp. fresh coriander leaves
- 2 or 3 green chilies finely chopped
- 1 ½ tbsp. lemon juice
- Salt and pepper to taste

INSTRUCTIONS

1. Blend the ingredients in a bowl and add water to it.
2. Preheat the Air Fryer to 160 F and cook for 25 minutes.
3. Continue turning them over to cook uniformly.
4. Serve either with mint chutney or ketchup.

85. White Lentil Galette

INGREDIENTS

- 2 cup white lentil soaked
- 3 tsp. ginger finely chopped
- 1-2 tbsp. fresh coriander leaves
- 2 or 3 green chilies finely chopped
- 1 ½ tbsp. lemon juice
- Salt and pepper to taste

INSTRUCTIONS

1. Wash the soaked lentils and mix it with the rest of the ingredients in a clean bowl.
2. Mold this mixture into round and flat galettes.
3. Wet the galettes slightly with water.
4. Preheat the Air Fryer to 160 F and cook for 25 minutes.
5. Serve either with mint chutney or ketchup.

86. Coconut and Plantain Pancakes

INGREDIENTS

- 2 fresh plantains (shredded)
- 1 cup shredded coconut
- 1 ½ cups almond flour
- 3 eggs
- 2 tsp. dried basil
- 2 tsp. dried parsley

- Salt and Pepper to taste
- 3 tbsp. Butter

INSTRUCTIONS

1. Preheat the air fryer to 250 F.
2. In a bowl, combine the ingredients. Mix well.
3. Cook till both sides of the pancake have browned. Serve with maple syrup.

87. Vegetable and Oat Muffins

INGREDIENTS

- 1 cup + 2 tbsp. whole wheat flour
- 1 ½ cup milk
- ½ tsp. baking powder
- ½ tsp. baking soda
- 2 tbsp. butter
- 1 cup + 3 tsp. sugar
- 3 tsp. vinegar
- ½ cup oats
- 1 cup mixed vegetables
- ½ tsp. vanilla essence
- Muffin cups or butter paper cups

INSTRUCTIONS

1. Combine the ingredients into a batter.
2. Pour into the muffin cups.
3. Preheat the fryer to 300 F and cook for 15 minutes.
4. Check whether the biscuits are cooked using a toothpick.

88. Vegan Avocado Fries

INGREDIENTS

- ½ cup breadcrumbs
- ½ tsp salt
- 1 Hass avocado
- aquafaba from 15 oz can of white beans

INSTRUCTIONS

1. In a major bowl, toss together the breadcrumbs and salt.
2. Empty the aquafaba into another shallow bowl.
3. Dip the avocado slices in the aquafaba and then in the breadcrumbs.

4. Air browning: Arrange the cuts in a single layer in your air fryer container.
5. Air fry for 10 minutes (Do not preheat) at 390F, shaking after 5 minutes.

89. Sweet Potato Chips

INGREDIENTS

- ½ tbsp tsp salt
- 3 sweet potatoes – peeled, washed and sliced
- ½ tsp dry pepper
- 2 tbsp of olive oil

INSTRUCTIONS

1. Place sliced sweet potatoes in a bowl. Add salt and dry pepper to mix with the potato.
2. Spread the olive oil over the mix.
3. Air fry at 370F for 20 minutes shaking after 10 minutes. Do not preheat.

90. Air Fryer Tofu Scramble

INGREDIENTS

- 1 block tofu
- 2 tbsp soy sauce
- 1 tsp garlic and onion powder
- 1/2 cup chopped onion
- 1 tsp turmeric
- 2 ½ cups chopped red potato
- 1 tbsp olive oil
- 4 cups broccoli florets

INSTRUCTIONS

1. Toss together the tofu, soy sauce, olive oil, turmeric, garlic powder, onion powder, and onion in a bowl.
2. In another bowl, toss the potatoes within the olive oil, and air fry at 400F for 15 minutes, shaking 7-8 minutes into cooking.
3. Add tofu after shaking the potatoes once more conserving any remaining marinade.
4. Cook the tofu and potatoes at 370F for 15 minutes.
5. Add broccoli to the air fryer for 5 minutes.

91. Avocado Egg Rolls and Sweet Chili Sauce
Servings: 5

INGREDIENTS

- 10 egg roll wrappers
- 3 avocados peeled and pitted
- 1 tomato, diced
- A pinch of salt and pepper
- coconut oil
- 4 tbsp sriracha
- 2 tbsp white sugar
- 1 tbsp rice vinegar
- 1 tbsp sesame oil

INSTRUCTIONS

1. Mash the avocados and mix in the ingredients. This will be the egg roll filling.
2. Dip the egg roll wrappers in a bowl of water.
3. Add filling onto the lower third of each wrapper.
4. Use your finger to brush water along the 4 edges of the wrapper.
5. Crease a corner over the filling, roll it up and seal. Repeat for each eggroll.
6. Add oil to a large skillet over medium heat. Cook for 3-5 minutes. Move to a paper towel to dry.
7. Combine sauce ingredients in a bowl and mix well.

92. Vegan Fried Ravioli
Servings: 4

INGREDIENTS

- 1/2 cup breadcrumbs
- 2 tsp nutritional yeast flakes
- 1 tsp dried basil
- 1 tsp dried oregano
- 1 tsp garlic powder
- Pinch salt & pepper
- 8 oz. thawed vegan ravioli
- Spritz cooking spray
- 1/2 cup marinara for dipping
- aquafaba

INSTRUCTIONS

1. Mix breadcrumbs, yeast flakes, dried basil, dried oregano, garlic powder, salt and pepper.
2. Put aquafaba into a bowl.

3. Dip ravioli into aquafaba, shake off extra fluid and coat in breadcrumbs.
4. Move the ravioli into the air fryer container. Set air fryer to 390 F and air fry for 6 minutes. Cautiously flip every ravioli over. Air fry for 2 additional minutes.
5. Remove ravioli from air fryer and serve with warm marinara sauce.

93. Air Fryer Cauliflower Chickpea Tacos
Servings: 4

INGREDIENTS

- 4 cups cauliflower florets
- 19 oz can of chickpeas
- 2 tbsp olive oil
- 2 tbsp taco seasoning
- 8 small tortillas
- 2 avocados sliced
- 4 cups cabbage shredded
- yogurt to drizzle

INSTRUCTIONS

1. Preheat air fryer to 390°F/200°C.
2. In a large bowl, toss the cauliflower and chickpeas with olive oil and taco flavoring.
3. Pour into the crate of your air fryer.
4. Cook for 20 minutes, or until cooked through.
5. Serve in tacos with avocado, cabbage, and yogurt.

94. Classic Falafel
Servings: 8

INGREDIENTS

- 1 ½ cups dry garbanzo beans
- ½ cup chopped fresh parsley
- 1/2 cup chopped fresh cilantro
- 1/2 cup chopped white onion
- 7 cloves garlic
- 2 Tbsp. All-purpose flour
- 1/2 tsp sea salt
- 1 Tbsp ground cumin
- 1/2 tbsp ground cardamom
- 1 tsp ground coriander
- 1/2 tbsp cayenne pepper

INSTRUCTIONS

1. Rinse garbanzo beans in a strainer and add to a large pot.
2. Cover with water and boil for 60 minutes. Drain completely.
3. In a food processor, mix parsley, cilantro, onions, and garlic.
4. Add garbanzo beans, flour, salt, cumin, cardamom, coriander and cayenne to food processor.
5. Place in a bowl, cover and refrigerate for 1-2 hours.
6. Remove from fridge and form into 1½-inch balls. Flatten slightly to create patties.
7. Preheat air fryer to 400° F. Add oil.
8. Place falafel into the container and cook for 10 minutes, turning partially through.

95. Thai Veggie Bites
Servings: 16

INGREDIENTS

- 1 Large Broccoli
- 1 Large Cauliflower
- 6 Large Carrots
- Handful Garden Peas
- ½ Cauliflower
- 1 Large Onion peeled and diced
- 1 Small Zucchini
- 2 Leeks cleaned and thinly sliced
- 1 Can Coconut Milk
- 50 g Plain Flour
- 1 cm Cube Ginger peeled and grated
- 1 Tbsp Garlic Puree
- 1 Tbsp Olive Oil
- 1 Tbsp Thai Green Curry Paste
- 1 Tbsp Coriander
- 1 Tbsp Mixed Spice
- 1 Tsp Cumin
- Salt & Pepper

INSTRUCTIONS

1. In a wok, cook the onion with the garlic, ginger and olive oil.
2. In a steamer, cook the vegetables (except the zucchini and leek) for 20 minutes.
3. Add the zucchini, leek and curry paste to the wok and cook over medium heat for a further 5 minutes.

4. Add the coconut milk and the rest of the seasoning. Mix well and then add the cauliflower rice.
5. Mix again and allow simmering for 10 minutes.
6. Add the steamed vegetables. Mix well.
7. Cool in the fridge for an hour.
8. Make into bite sized pieces and place in the Air Fryer. Cook for 10 minutes at 180 C.

96. Garlic and Herb Air-Fryer Roasted Chickpeas
Servings: 4

INGREDIENTS

- 2 cans of chickpeas
- 1 tbsp olive oil
- 1 tbsp nutritional yeast
- 2 tsp garlic powder
- 1 tbsp mixed herbs (rosemary, thyme, and oregano)
- Sea salt and black pepper to taste

INSTRUCTIONS

1. Drain and wash the chickpeas. Add to a medium-sized bowl with the olive oil and seasonings.
2. Preheat air fryer to 200° C and bake for 15-20 minutes, shaking once at the 10-minute mark.
3. Serve warm.

97. Spicy Cauliflower Stir-Fry
Servings: 4

INGREDIENTS

- 1 head cauliflower
- 3/4 cup onion white
- 5 cloves garlic
- 1 1/2 tsp tamari
- 1 tbsp rice vinegar
- 1/2 tsp coconut sugar
- 1 tbsp Sriracha
- 2 scallions for garnish

INSTRUCTIONS

1. Set the air fryer temperature to 350 F. Cook the cauliflower for 10 minutes.
2. Add the cut onion, mix and cook 10 additional minutes.
3. Add garlic, mix and cook 5 additional minutes.

4. Mix soy sauce, rice vinegar, coconut sugar, Sriracha, salt, and pepper together in a little bowl.
5. Add the blend to cauliflower and mix. Cook 5 more minutes.
6. To serve, garnish with cut scallions.

98. Vegan Corn Fritters
Servings: 5

INGREDIENTS

- 2 C of Fresh Frozen Corn Kernels
- 1 C of Corn + 2-3 Tbsp Almond Milk
- 1/3 C Finely Ground Cornmeal
- 1/3 C Flour
- 1/2 tsp Salt
- 1/4 tsp Pepper
- 1/2 tsp Baking Powder
- Onion Powder
- Garlic Powder
- 1/4 tsp Paprika
- 2 Tbsp Green Chiles with juices
- About 1/4 C Italian Parsley
- Vegetable Oil

INSTRUCTIONS

1. Combine all dry ingredients.
2. In a food processor, mix 1 cup of corn with 2-3 Tbsp. of almond milk, salt and pepper.
3. Add the corn blend to the dry ingredients and mix.
4. Add corn kernels.
5. Preheat a skillet over medium-high heat with 1 Tbsp of oil.
6. Cook on one side until golden brown and flip, cooking the opposite side.
7. Mix the sauce ingredients and serve.

99. Crispy Seasoned Jicama Fries
Servings: 4

INGREDIENTS

- 1 lb. jicama
- 3 tbsp butter or oil
- 1 tbsp chili powder
- 1-2 tsp salt, to taste
- 1/2 tsp garlic powder
- 1/2 tsp onion powder
- dash of paprika

- dash of black pepper

INSTRUCTIONS

1. Preheat stove to 400 F.
2. Peel and cut jicama into French fry shapes. Boil for 15 minutes. Remove and pat dry.
3. Mix together butter/oil and seasonings.
4. Toss jicama in flavoring blend till uniformly coated.
5. Spread in a single layer on a baking sheet and bake for 40 minutes, flipping part of the way through.

100. Air Fryer Plantains

Servings: 2

INGREDIENTS

- 1 plantain
- 3/4 tsp oil
- 1/2 tbsp of salt

INSTRUCTIONS

1. Peel the plantain and cut into slices.
2. Add salt to taste
3. Sprinkle oil on the plantain
4. Place inside the air fryer preheated to 360 F for 3 minutes per side.

101. Air Fryer Green Bean and Mushroom Casserole

Servings: 6

INGREDIENTS

- 24 oz. fresh green beans
- 2 cups sliced button mushrooms
- 1 fresh lemon – juiced
- 1 tbsp garlic powder
- 3/4 tsp ground sage
- 1 tsp onion powder
- 3/4 tsp salt
- 3/4 tsp black pepper
- Oil spray
- Any type of fries

INSTRUCTIONS

1. In a large bowl, mix green beans, mushrooms, lemon juice, garlic powder, sage, onion powder, salt, and pepper.
2. Air fry at 400 F for 10-12 minutes, shaking each 2-3 minutes.
3. Serve with French seared onions.

102. Air Fryer Buffalo Cauliflower

Servings: 4

INGREDIENTS

- 4 cups cauliflower florets
- 1 cup breadcrumbs
- 1 tsp sea salt
- 1/4 cup melted vegan butter
- 1/4 cup vegan Buffalo sauce
- vegan mayo – Cashew Ranch, any creamy salad dressing

INSTRUCTIONS

1. Melt the vegan butter.
2. Holding by the stem, plunge each floret into the vegan Buffalo sauce.
3. Hold the florets over a bowl until trickling of sauce stops.
4. Dip the florets in the breadcrumb/salt mixture.
5. Air fry at 350 F for 14-17 minutes, shaking a couple of times.
6. Serve with any dipping sauce of choice.

103. Air Fryer Brussels Sprouts

Servings: 2 servings

INGREDIENTS

- 2 cups Brussels sprouts (sliced)
- 1 tbsp olive oil
- 1 tbsp balsamic vinegar
- 1/4 tsp sea salt

INSTRUCTIONS

1. In a bowl, toss together the Brussels, oil, and salt.
2. Air fry at 400 F for 8-10 minutes, shaking after 5 minutes.

104.   Crunchy Breadcrumb Tofu
Servings: 4

INGREDIENTS

- 1 block extra firm tofu
- 1 tbsp toasted sesame oil
- 1/4 cup soy sauce
- 1 tsp rice vinegar
- 1/2 tsp garlic powder
- 1 tsp ground ginger
- 1/2 cup vegan mayo
- 1 cup breadcrumbs
- 1 tsp sea salt

INSTRUCTIONS

1. In a small bowl, whisk together the sesame oil, soy sauce, vinegar, garlic powder, and ginger.
2. Add the vegetarian mayo.
3. In another bowl, whisk the breadcrumb and salt.
4. Dip each tofu piece into the mayo, then the breadcrumb combo.
5. Arrange the pieces in a single layer.
6. Cook at 370 F for 20 minutes, shaking delicately following 10 minutes

105.   Air Fryer Sushi Rolls
Servings: 3

INGREDIENTS

- 1 1/2 cups chopped kale
- 1/2 tsp rice vinegar
- 3/4 tsp toasted sesame oil
- 1/8 tsp garlic powder
- 1/4 tsp ground ginger
- 3/4 tsp soy sauce
- 1 tbsp sesame seeds
- For the Kale Salad Sushi Rolls
- 1 batch Pressure Cooker Sushi Rice
- 3 sheets of sushi nori
- 1/2 of a Hass avocado – sliced
- 1/4 cup vegan mayonnaise
- sriracha sauce
- 1/2 cup breadcrumbs

INSTRUCTIONS

1. Mix the kale, vinegar, sesame oil, garlic powder, ground ginger, and soy sauce.

2. Mix in the sesame seeds and set aside.
3. Lay out a sheet of nori. Spread a thin layer of rice onto the nori.
4. Spread 2-3 tbsp of the kale mixture and top with avocado.
5. Wrap the sushi roll, squeezing delicately to get a nice, tight roll. Seal the seam shut with water.
6. With 3 more sushi rolls.
7. In a shallow bowl, whisk together the veggie lover mayo with sriracha.
8. Pour the breadcrumbs into a shallow bowl.
9. Coat sushi rolls in the Sriracha Mayo, then the breadcrumbs.
10. Air fry at 390 F for 10 minutes, shaking tenderly following 5 minutes.
11. Cut each roll into 6-8 pieces.
12. Serve with soy sauce for dipping.

106.   Air Fryer Jackfruit Taquitos
Preparation Time: 30 minutes
Servings: 2

INGREDIENTS

- 14 oz. water-packed jackfruit
- 1 cup cooked or canned red beans
- 1/2 cup pico de gallo sauce
- 1/4 cup plus 2 tbsp water
- 4 6-inch corn
- 4 spritzes canola oil

INSTRUCTIONS

1. In a medium pan, combine the jackfruit, beans, pico de gallo, and water.
2. Using a pan, heat the jackfruit blend over medium-high heat.
3. Decrease the heat and stew for 20 to 25 minutes.
4. Mash the jackfruit blend with a fork or potato masher to a substantial surface.
5. Preheat the air fryer to 370 F for 3 minutes.
6. Place a tortilla on a work surface. Spoon 1/4 cup of the jackfruit blend onto the tortilla.
7. Repeat this procedure to make 4 taquitos.
8. Spritz the air fryer crate with the oil. Place the folded tortillas into the air fryer.
9. Cook at 370 F for 8 minutes.

107.   Garlicky Roasted Almonds
Servings: 8

INGREDIENTS

- 1 tbsp soy sauce
- 1 tbsp garlic powder
- 1 tsp paprika
- 1/4 tsp pepper
- 2 cups raw almonds

INSTRUCTIONS

1. In a large bowl, mix ingredients, with the exception of the almonds, to form a thick paste. Mix in the almonds.
2. Transfer the almonds to your air fryer bin, and cook at 320 for 6-8 minutes, shaking at regular intervals to cook uniformly.
3. Starting at minute 6, you'll need to check in consistently, tasting almond for doneness. Let them cool to room temperature around 10-15 minutes

108. Air Fryer Hush Puppies
Servings: 4

INGREDIENTS

- 1 cup cornmeal
- 1 1/2 tsp of baking powder
- 1/2 tsp salt
- 1/4 cup soy milk
- 1 tsp apple cider vinegar
- 1/4 cup minced onion
- 1/4 cup aquafaba
- 1 tbsp vegan sugar
- 1 tbsp olive oil
- spray oil

INSTRUCTIONS

1. Mix the cornmeal, baking powder and salt in a medium-sized bowl.
2. Mix in the milk, apple cider vinegar, onion, aquafaba, sugar and olive oil.
3. Form small balls and place in the air fryer container.
4. Cook at 390°F for 10 minutes.

109. Lemon Tofu Piccata
Servings: 4

INGREDIENTS

- 1/4 cup fresh lemon juice
- 2 tbsp parsley
- 1 clove garlic
- 1/2 tsp sea salt
- 1/2 tsp black pepper

For the Tofu:

- 1 block extra firm tofu – pressed and cut into 8 rectangular cutlets
- 1/2 cup vegan mayo
- 1 cup breadcrumbs
- 1/4 cup lemon juice
- 1 cup vegetable broth
- 2 tbsp parsley
- 1 clove garlic
- 2 tsp potato starch or cornstarch
- 1/2 tsp sea salt
- 1/4 tsp black pepper
- 2 tbsp capers
- 1 lemon sliced into rounds

INSTRUCTIONS

1. Combine the marinade ingredients in a blender or food processor.
2. Marinate the tofu for 15-30 minutes.
3. In a small bowl, whisk together the sesame oil, soy sauce, vinegar, garlic powder, and ginger.
4. Add the vegan mayo.
5. In another bowl, whisk the breadcrumb and salt.
6. Dip each tofu piece into the mayo, then the breadcrumb combo.
7. Arrange the pieces in a single layer.
8. Cook at 370 F for 20 minutes, shaking delicately after 10 minutes.
9. While the tofu cooks, combine the sauce ingredients in a blender or food processor.
10. Puree until smooth.
11. Pour the sauce into a pan. Simmer for 5-7 minutes, until it thickens.

110. Vegan Mashed Potato Bowl
Servings: 4

INGREDIENTS

- 3 large red potatoes - cut into pieces and cooked with the skin on.

- 2 tbsp vegan butter
- 1/2 cup unsweetened soy milk
- Salt and black pepper
- 1 block extra firm tofu - pressed and cut into pieces
- 2 tbsp soy sauce
- 1 tsp garlic powder
- 1 tbsp olive oil
- 4 packed cups chopped kale
- 1 cup fresh or frozen corn kernels
- 1 tsp garlic powder
- 2 tbsp seasoned rice vinegar

INSTRUCTIONS

1. Preheat the stove to 425 F.
2. Boil and mash the potatoes with the soy milk.
3. Cover the bowl, and set aside.
4. Make the Tofu While the Potatoes Cook.
5. Place the tofu in a single layer to your air fryer crate, and sprinkle with soy sauce and garlic powder, being positive to cowl the entirety of the tofu.
6. Air fry at 400F for 20 minutes, shaking the subsequent 10 minutes.
7. Cook the Kale and Corn when the Tofu has 10 Minutes remaining.
8. Heat the oil in a large griddle over medium-high heat.
9. Add the kale and corn, and sprinkle with garlic powder.
10. Cook, blending, till the kale begins to wither, 4-5 minutes.
11. Add the rice vinegar, mixing to cover the greens and corn.

111. Vegan Breakfast Sandwich
Servings: 4

INGREDIENTS

- 1 block extra firm tofu
- 1/4 cup light soy sauce
- 1 tsp garlic powder
- 1/2 tsp turmeric
- Dash of paprika
- 4 vegan English muffins
- Vegan mayonnaise
- 1 Hass avocado
- 4 slices your favorite vegan cheese
- Sliced onion
- Sliced tomato

INSTRUCTIONS

1. Mix marinade ingredients and marinate tofu for 10 minutes.
2. Place the tofu in a single layer in air fryer crate, and sprinkle with soy sauce and garlic powder.
3. Air fry at 400F for 20 minutes, shaking after 10 minutes.
4. Make the Sandwich. Spread your English muffins with vegan mayo.
5. Add the avocado, vegan cheese, and ingredients of your choice.

112. Ginger Tofu Vegan Sushi Bowl

Servings: 4

INGREDIENTS

- 2-piece fresh ginger
- 1 clove garlic
- 2 tbsp maple syrup
- 1 tbsp toasted sesame oil
- 2 tbsp soy sauce
- 1 tsp rice vinegar
- 1 tbsp cornstarch
- 1 block extra firm tofu
- 1/2 cup carrot sticks
- 3/4 cup cucumber
- 1 Hass avocado
- 16 oz of roasted seaweed snacks
- 1/4 cup pickled ginger
- 1/2 cup roasted cashews
- 1 green onion

INSTRUCTIONS

1. To make the marinade, combine the ginger, garlic, maple syrup, sesame oil, soy sauce, and vinegar in your blender or food processor.
2. Puree until smooth.
3. In a large bowl, toss together the tofu and the marinade.
4. Put aside to marinate for 10 minutes. Drain any extra marinade.
5. Toss the marinated tofu with cornstarch in a similar bowl and place in the air fryer.
6. Cook on 370F for 15 minutes, shaking after 8 minutes.
7. Top with tofu, avocado, green onion, carrots, cucumbers, seaweed snacks, and cured ginger.

8. Sprinkle on the cashews. Garnish with green onion.

113. Air Fryer Baby Bok Choy
Servings: 4

INGREDIENTS

- 4 bunches baby bok choy
- Spray oil
- 1 tsp garlic powder

INSTRUCTIONS

1. Cut the bottoms off of washed bok choy bunches, and separate the leaves.
2. Place in the air fryer, lightly coated in oil. Sprinkle on the garlic powder.
3. Bake at 350F for 5-6 minutes, shaking after 2 minutes

114. Air Fryer Roasted Butternut Squash
Servings: 6

INGREDIENTS

- 4 cups diced butternut squash
- 1 cup sliced green onions
- 8 oz. button mushrooms
- 1 tbsp olive oil
- 1 tbsp balsamic vinegar
- 1 tbsp soy sauce
- 1 tbsp maple syrup
- 4 cloves fresh garlic
- 1/4 cup dried cranberries
- Extra green onion

INSTRUCTIONS

1. In a large bowl, mix the squash, green onions, and mushrooms, and set aside.
2. Combine the olive oil, soy sauce, maple syrup, vinegar, and garlic in your blender or food processor, and puree until smooth.
3. Pour the sauce over the squash blend, tossing to cover well.
4. Place in air fryer and cook at 400F for 25-35 minutes, shaking at regular intervals.
5. Toss in dried cranberries, top with the additional green onion.

115. Oat Cutlet
Servings: 4

INGREDIENTS

- 1/2 cup of boiled rice
- 1/4 cup of soaked and drained oats (5 min)
- 1/4 cup of beaten rice
- 1 sliced onion
- chopped coriander leaves 1-2 stems
- 1 tsp black or black salt

INSTRUCTIONS

1. Mix all the ingredients.
2. Create little balls with the dough and flatten.
3. Put in the air fryer for 10-15 minutes at 200.

116. Banana Chips
Servings: 2

INGREDIENTS

- 4 raw green bananas
- 1/2 tbsp Black pepper
- 1/2 tbsp Salt
- Oil

INSTRUCTIONS

1. Peel the Banana and slice into thin chips
2. Add little or no oil to the chips
3. Air fry for 10 minutes at 180C.
4. Add salt and pepper to taste.

117. Crispy Potato Cheese Balls
Servings: 4

INGREDIENTS

- 2-3 Boiled, mashed potatoes
- Chopped capsicum
- Coriander leaves and green chili
- 1tbsp ginger and garlic paste
- 3 tbsp of corn flour
- 3 tbsp of flour
- 1 tbsp salt, oregano and red chili flakes
- 1 cup of breadcrumbs
- Small cube size chess pieces

INSTRUCTIONS

1. In A bowl add chopped capsicum, coriander leaves and green chili to the mashed potatoes
2. Add garlic paste, 2 tbsp flour and 1 tbsp corn flour to the mixed potatoes earlier and make small balls.
3. Take small cheese cubes and press them inside these balls and give it a round shape.
4. Add 1 tbsp of all-purpose flour and 1tbsp corn and 1/2 cup of water to matter a batter.
5. Dip the balls in this batter and then roll over breadcrumbs
6. Prepare these balls in the refrigerator for 30 minutes before cooking.
7. Air fry these balls for 10-15 minutes at 200C.

118. Air Fryer Roasted Chana

Servings: 2

INGREDIENTS

- 1 tsp salt
- Spray oil
- 100gms chana
- 1 tsp black pepper

INSTRUCTIONS

1. Boil 100gms of chana with 1 tsp salt for 5 minutes.
2. Drain the water and spray with oil
3. Air fry for 10 minutes at 180C

119. Cheese Spinach Balls

Servings: 2

INGREDIENTS

- 300gms Spinach leaves
- 1 cup Breadcrumbs
- Grated Mozzarella cheese
- Red chili flakes
- Chopped onion
- Corn flour
- Grated garlic
- 1 tsp Salt
- Oil

INSTRUCTIONS

1. Make spinach puree utilizing paste of spinach leaves with breadcrumbs, ground mozzarella, corn flour, garlic, and salt and form into little balls.
2. Mix cheese, chili flakes, and onions and form into little balls, place them inside the spinach balls.
3. Brush them with oil
4. Air fry at 200C for 10-15 minutes.
5. Serve hot and fresh with red tomato sauce.

120. Poppy Seed Cutlet

Servings: 5

INGREDIENTS

- 1 Boiled Potato
- 1/2 cup white poppy seeds
- 1 green chili
- 1 small onion
- 1/2 tsp salt

INSTRUCTIONS

1. Dry grind the poppy seeds in a mixer
2. Wet grind to form paste.
3. Add all other ingredients to this paste and form small cutlets using the palm of your hands.
4. Refrigerate for 30 minutes.
5. Brush with oil and air fry for 10 minutes at 200C. Air fry again at 160C for 5 minutes.
6. Serve hot

121. Pani Puri

Servings: 2

INGREDIENTS

- 1 cup of pani puri chips
- 1/2 tbsp salt
- Oil

INSTRUCTIONS

1. Add salt to the chips to taste.
2. Preheat the Air fryer for 5 minutes at 200C.
3. Place the chips in the air fryer for 2 minutes at 200C.
4. Serve

122. Crispy Cheese Potato Cutlet

Servings: 3

INGREDIENTS

- 3 medium size Potato
- 2 cubes Mozzarella Cheese
- 1/2 cup Breadcrumbs
- 1 tbsp Olive Oil
- 1 tsp Salt
- 1 pc Green Chili
- 4 pieces Garlic clove
- 1 tsp Oregano
- 1 tsp chaat masala

INSTRUCTIONS

1. Mash the potatoes with all ingredients except breadcrumbs.
2. Make small cutlets and coat with breadcrumbs.
3. Air fry for 10 minutes at 180C and then 5 minutes at 200 C.
4. Serve hot with a dipping sauce.

123. Air Fryer Pineapple

Servings: 2

INGREDIENTS

- Pineapple, chopped
- 1/2 salt

INSTRUCTIONS

1. Sprinkle the sliced pineapple with salt.
2. Put it in the air fryer for 10 minutes at 160C
3. Serve

124. Paneer and Cheese Veg Keto Cutlet

Servings: 3

INGREDIENTS

- 2 cups of Cottage Cheese
- 1 cup of grated pizza cheese
- 1 finely chopped onion
- 1/2 tsp garlic powder
- 1/2 tsp chaat masala
- 1/2 tsp salt
- 1/2 tsp oregano seasoning
- 1 tsp butter

INSTRUCTIONS

1. Mix all the ingredients in a bowl
2. Make little cutlets of any form you want
3. Place them inside the air fryer and air fryer at 180C for 10 minutes.

125. Cheese Paneer Balls

Servings: 4

INGREDIENTS

- 200gm grated Indian cottage cheese
- Cheese diced into cubes
- 2 tbsp Gram flour
- 1 tbsp Corn flour
- 2 Finely chopped onion
- 1 Finely chopped green chili
- Finely chopped ginger
- 1/3 tsp Red chili powder
- Chopped coriander leaves
- Cooking oil
- 1/2 tsp Salt

INSTRUCTIONS

1. Mix all the ingredients into the paneer except cheese and oil.
2. Form a small portion of mixture into a ball and flatten.
3. Stuff one cheese cube inside, seal the edges and make a ball by rolling it on your palm.
4. Repeat till mixture is finished
5. Air fry the balls for 10-15 minutes at 200C.
6. Serve hot.

126. Bati Chokha

INGREDIENTS

Bati:

- Wheat flour, ajwain, salt, ghee

For Stuffing:

- Roasted gram flour
- Green chilies
- Dhaniya leaves
- Roasted jeera,
- garlic, amchur, mango pickle masala, lemon juice

- onions, mustard oil, salt to taste

For Chokha:

- Boiled potatoes
- Salt

For Chutney:

- Garlic
- Red chili
- Mustard seeds and Ghee

INSTRUCTIONS

1. Mix the flour and salt, ajwain, kalonji, and oil. Set aside for 20 minutes
2. For stuffing: combine ingredients: in a bowl.
3. Sprinkle some water to guarantee that the stuffing is not excessively dry
4. For bati: mix ingredients and make 6 to7 balls from the mixture.
5. Fill each with stuffing and close the balls around it.
6. Brush them with oil and air fry for 15 minutes at 200 C.
7. For chokha: mixture potatoes and tomatoes, encompass finely hacked onion, coriander leaves, salt, green chilies, and oil. Include all the ingredients.
8. For the chutney: crush all ingredients: apart from ghee and mustard seeds. & later on, sauté the paste in ghee and mustard.

127. Paneer Tikka

INGREDIENTS

- Paneer 200g cubed
- Onion 25g cubed
- Tomato 25g cubed
- Capsicum 25g cubed
- Hung curd 50g
- Corn flour 10g
- Ginger garlic paste 5g
- Cream 10mL
- Cumin powder ¼ tsp
- Red chili powder ½ tsp
- Oil For brushing
- Salt and Pepper To taste
- Long Toothpicks – 15-20 pieces

INSTRUCTIONS

1. In a bowl, blend hung curd, corn flour, ginger-garlic paste, cream, cumin powder, red chili powder, salt and pepper to make the marinade.
2. Put the paneer and vegetable cubes into the marinade and coat well. Set aside for 30 minutes.
3. Preheat the air fryer to 180 C for 5 minutes. Brush the wire rack with oil.
4. Place the paneer tikka strung onto toothpicks in the Air fryer and air fry for 5 minutes.
5. Serve hot with the choice of serving of mixed greens and chutney

128. Nutty French Toast
Servings 8

INGREDIENTS

- 1 cup rolled oats
- 1 cup pecan nut
- 2 tbsp ground flax seed
- 1 tsp ground cinnamon
- 8 pieces whole grain vegan bread
- 1 cup nondairy milk
- Maple syrup

INSTRUCTIONS

1. Add oats, nuts, flaxseed and cinnamon to a food processor and blend till it looks like breadcrumbs.
2. Pour into a pan and dip bread slices in.
3. Add the milk to another bowl and soak bread in milk for about 15 seconds on each side.
4. Place coated bread in air fryer basket without overlapping.
5. Cook at 180° C for 3 minutes, flip and cook for another 3 minutes.
6. Repeat for all the bread until coated and cooked.
7. Serve with maple syrup and enjoy.

129. Air Fryer Tofu Rancheros
Servings: 4

INGREDIENTS

- 1 container super firm tofu, cut into cubes
- 1 tsp ground cumin powder

- 1 tsp ground chili powder
- 1/2 tsp paprika
- Salt to taste

INSTRUCTIONS

1. Preheat air fryer to 200°C.
2. Toss tofu cubes in cumin, chili powder, paprika and salt.
3. Add coated tofu to air fryer basket.
4. Cook for 5 minutes, shake basket and cook for another 5 minutes.
5. Serve with veggies.

130. Air Fryer Chips

Total time: 30 minutes
Servings: 2

INGREDIENTS

- 2 large red potatoes
- 2 tbsp vegan parmesan cheese
- 2 tsp salt
- 4 minced garlic cloves

INSTRUCTIONS

1. Slice potatoes thinly and place in a bowl of water.
2. Add 2 tsp salt and allow to soak and absorb for 30 minutes.
3. Drain and pat dry with paper towels.
4. Toss moist potatoes with garlic and parmesan.
5. Place potatoes in air fryer basket but don't overload.
6. Fry at 90° C for 20 to 25 minutes. Toss basket and fry for another 5 minutes.
7. Increase temperature to 200°C and fry for another 5 minutes or until crunchy.
8. Enjoy your snack!

131. Chickpeas with Tandoori Spice

Total time: 15 minutes
Servings: 3

INGREDIENTS

- 1 can chickpeas, rinsed and drained
- 1 tbsp olive oil
- 2 tsp tandoori sauce or any spice blend of your choice
- 1/2 tbsp salt

INSTRUCTIONS

1. Preheat air fryer to 200° C
2. In a bowl, combine chickpeas with olive oil, salt and spices
3. Arrange in a single layer at bottom of air fryer and cook for 8 to 10 minutes, shaking basket halfway through.
4. Remove and allow to cool.
5. Repeat for the remaining chickpeas.

132. Air Fryer Ravioli

Total time: 25 minutes
Servings: 4

INGREDIENTS

- 2 tsp nutritional yeast
- 1 tsp dried basil
- 1/2 cup breadcrumbs
- 1 tsp garlic powder
- 1 tsp dried oregano
- 1/4 cup aquafaba
- 8 oz. thawed vegan ravioli
- Salt and pepper to taste

INSTRUCTIONS

1. Combine breadcrumbs, yeast drops, basil, oregano, garlic powder, salt and pepper on a plate.
2. Pour aquafaba in a bowl.
3. First dunk ravioli in aquafaba, then in breadcrumb blend. Coat uniformly.
4. Transfer ravioli to air fryer.
5. Spray with a cooking oil and air fry at 200 ° C for 6 minutes.
6. Flip and cook for an additional 2 minutes.
7. Serve with warm marinara.

133. Crispy Tater Tots

Total time: 25 minutes
Servings: 12

INGREDIENTS

- 1 cup sweet potato puree
- 1/4 tsp cumin
- 1/4 tsp salt
- 1/4 cup breadcrumbs
- 1/4 tsp coriander
- Cooking spray

INSTRUCTIONS

1. Preheat air to 200° C.
2. Mix all ingredients in a bowl.
3. Scoop and form into tots; arrange on a plate.
4. Spray tots with oil.
5. Cook in air fryer for 6 to 7 minutes, flip and continue for 6 to 7 more minutes.
6. Serve warm with ketchup.

134.   Air Fryer Popcorn Tofu

Total time: 30 minutes
Servings: 4

INGREDIENTS

- 14 oz. Super firm tofu, pressed and drained
- 1/2 cup cornmeal
- 1/2 cup chickpea flour
- 2 tbsp nutritional yeast
- 1 tbsp better-than bouillon no chicken base
- 1 tbsp Dijon mustard
- 1 tsp garlic powder and onion powder
- 1/2 tsp salt and pepper
- 1 cup unsweetened dairy free milk
- 1 1/2 cups breadcrumbs

INSTRUCTIONS

1. Place all ingredients aside from tofu and breadcrumbs in a large bowl and combine.
2. Place breadcrumbs in another bowl.
3. Dip tofu into the batter, then in breadcrumbs.
4. Place in air fryer bin and cook at 175° C for 12 minutes, shaking container part way through.
5. Serve with mayo and sriracha.

135.   Air Fryer Soy Curls

Total time: 25 minutes
Servings: 2

INGREDIENTS

- 4 oz. Butler soy curls
- 1/4 cup nutritional yeast
- 1 tsp poultry seasoning
- 1/4 cup finely ground cornmeal
- 2 tsp Cajun seasoning
- 3 cups boiling water

INSTRUCTIONS

1. Put soy twists in a dish and pour water on them. Permit to soak for 8 minutes.
2. Drain and press extra water out with a large spoon.
3. Mix the remaining ingredients in a bowl and consist of depleted twists into the bowl to cover nicely.
4. Place in an air fryer and cook at 190° C for 5 minutes.
5. Shake and cook for an extra 5 minutes.
6. Serve with pureed potatoes.

136.   Spring Rolls

Total time: 30 minutes
Servings: 4

INGREDIENTS

- 3 tbsp tamari
- 2 tsp liquid smoke
- 2 tbsp cashew butter
- 4 pieces of rice paper
- 2 cups tofu scramble
- 8 strips roasted red pepper
- 7 stalks asparagus
- 1 small broccoli
- 1/3 cup sweet potatoes, diced
- Spinach, kale or other greens

INSTRUCTIONS

1. Pre-warm temperature air fryer to 175° C and line container with wax paper.
2. In a bowl, whisk cashew butter, tamari, water, and liquid smoke.
3. Prepare a working space for the rice paper.
4. Dip rice paper under running water and hydrate for 5-10 seconds.
5. Place tofu and veggies inside rice paper and roll up.
6. Plunge each roll into the cashew combo and coat liberally.
7. Transfer to the coated air fryer bin and air fry for 15 minutes.
8. Flip and proceed for a further 10 minutes.

137.   Vegan Onion Rings

Total time: 40 minutes
Servings: 6

INGREDIENTS

- 3 medium yellow onions

Wet mix:

- 1/2 tsp paprika
- 1/2 tsp salt
- 1/4 tsp turmeric powder
- 2/3 cup unsweetened nondairy milk
- 1/2 cup all-purpose flour

Dry mix:

- 1 cup breadcrumbs
- 1/2 tsp paprika
- 1/4 tsp turmeric
- 1/4 tsp salt

INSTRUCTIONS

1. Preheat air fryer to 200°C.
2. Remove the onion skin. Cut into 1/2-inch round slices.
3. Place all wet ingredients in a bowl and mix well.
4. Place all dry ingredients in another bowl and blend.
5. Dunk onion rings in the wet blend, then in the dry blend. Cover uniformly with breadcrumbs.
6. Place in air fryer bin and air fry for 8 to 10 minutes.

138. Air Fryer Wontons

Total time: 25 minutes
Servings: 30

INGREDIENTS

- 30 wonton wrappers
- 1/2 cup onion, grated
- 1 tbsp chili sauce
- 1/2 tsp white pepper
- 1 cup grated cabbage
- 1/2 cup grated carrots
- 1/2 cup finely chopped mushrooms
- 1/2 cup finely chopped red pepper
- Pinch of salt

INSTRUCTIONS

1. In a saucepan, heat all vegetables and cook until moisture from mushrooms is released.
2. Remove from heat and stir in chili sauce, garlic powder, white pepper and salt. Allow to cool.
3. Place a wonton wrapper on your working table and add 1 tbsp veggie mixture to the center of the wrapper.
4. Run wet finger along the exposed top of the wrapper and carefully pull the bottom over the mixture.
5. Wet finger again and wet the bottom corners of wonton.
6. Gently fold over the bottom corners of wonton so one sits on the top of another and seal with light pressure.
7. Repeat for remaining wonton wrappers and place in preheated air fryer.
8. Spray with cooking spray.
9. Air fry at 160° C for 6 minutes or until golden brown.
10. Allow to cool before serving with soy sauce or any dipping sauce of your choice.

139. Air Fryer Vegan Tempeh Bacon

Total time: 20
Servings: 5

INGREDIENTS

- 4oz organic Tempeh, sliced thin
- 1/2 tbsp Liquid Smoke
- 1 tsp oil
- 1/4 cup low-sodium soy sauce
- 1/4 tsp black pepper
- 1/4 tsp garlic powder
- 1/4 tsp paprika
- 1 tbsp maple syrup

INSTRUCTIONS

1. Combine marinade ingredients in a shallow bowl and marinate tempeh cuts for 10 minutes, flipping over partway through.
2. Line the base of your air fryer bin with parchment paper.
3. Place tempeh in the fry bin and sprinkle with more marinade.
4. Air fry at 175°C for 10 minutes, flipping part of the way through and grease remaining marinade over cuts.

140. Kale and Potato Nuggets

Total time: 50 minutes
Servings: 4

INGREDIENTS

- 2 cups chopped potatoes
- 1/8 cup almond milk
- 1 clove minced garlic
- 4 cups coarsely chopped kale
- 1 tsp extra-virgin olive oil
- 1/4 tsp sea salt
- 1/8 tsp ground black pepper
- Vegetable oil spray

INSTRUCTIONS

1. Boil potatoes for 20 minutes.
2. In a pan, warm oil and sauté garlic. Add kale and cook for 2 to 3 minutes. Move to a bowl.
3. Drain potatoes and mash them in a bowl with milk, pepper, and salt. Mix with the cooked kale.
4. Preheat the air fryer to 200° C for 5 minutes.
5. Roll potato and kale blend into 1-inch chunks. Splash air fryer field with vegetable oil. Air fry for 12 to 15 minutes, shaking at 6 minutes.
6. Serve and respect it.

141. Air Fryer Eggplant Parmesan

Servings:

INGREDIENTS

- 1 large eggplant, sliced
- 1 cup all-purpose flour
- 1/2 cup almond milk
- 2 tbsp vegan parmesan cheese
- 1/4 cup vegan parmesan
- 1 tbsp fresh parsley
- 1/2 cup breadcrumbs
- Olive oil cooking spray

INSTRUCTIONS

1. Coat eggplant in flour, then in almond milk lastly in parmesan breadcrumbs.
2. Transfer eggplant into air fryer basket and splash with cooking oil.
3. Air fry at 175°C for 15 minutes, flipping part of the way through.

4. Top with some marinara sauce and vegan parmesan and air fry for an additional 2 minutes.
5. Garnish with crisp parsley and serve with pasta or more marinara sauce.

142. Portobello Mushroom Pizza

Total time: 25 minutes
Servings: 4

INGREDIENTS

- 4 large portobello mushrooms, washed and de-stemmed and de-gilled
- salt and black pepper
- 4 tbsp oil-free pasta sauce
- balsamic vinegar
- 1 clove garlic, minced
- 3 oz. zucchini, chopped
- 2 tbsp diced sweet red pepper
- 4 kalamata olives, sliced
- 1 tsp dried basil
- Fresh basil leaves, minced

INSTRUCTIONS

1. Pat the internal components of portobello dry and splash the 2 sides with balsamic vinegar.
2. Sprinkle with salt and pepper.
3. Spread 1 tbsp of pasta sauce internal each mushroom and sprinkle with garlic.
4. Preheat Air Fryer to 165°C.
5. Place mushrooms in a single layer into the air fryer basket.
6. Air Fry for 6 minutes, flipping halfway through.

143. Air Fryer Donuts

Total time: 18 minutes
Servings: 4

INGREDIENTS

Coating:

- 1/2 cup melted vegan butter
- 2 tbsp cinnamon
- 1 cup sugar

Donut:

- 1 cup gluten free cereal
- 2 tbsp sugar

- 1/2 cup nondairy milk
- 1/4 cup vegetable shortening
- 1/2 tsp salt
- 1 tbsp baking powder
- 1 1/2 cup gluten free flour

INSTRUCTIONS

1. Pour melted butter into a bowl, then add sugar and cinnamon and set aside.
2. In a bowl, mix cereal, flour, sugar, baking powder and salt. Fold in shortening.
3. Roll mixture into medium balls.
4. Place donut holes in air fryer basket and air fry at 190°C for 6 minutes, shaking basket halfway through.
5. Carefully dip donut holes into coating mixture.

144.   Air Fryer Chex Mix

Total time: 16 minutes
Servings: 6

INGREDIENTS

- 2 cups rice Chex cereals
- 2 cups corn Chex cereals
- 1 cup pretzels
- 1/4 cup pumpkin seeds
- 3 tbsp butter, vegan
- 1 tbsp garlic salt

INSTRUCTIONS

1. In a bowl, combine rice Chex, corn Chex, pumpkin seeds, and pretzels.
2. Melt butter and pour over your blend. Add garlic salt, mix together to cover.
3. Air fry at 175°C for 3 minutes, shake crate and air fry for an additional 2 minutes.

145.   Air Fryer Broccoli

Total time: 12 minutes
Servings: 2

INGREDIENTS

- 3 cups broccoli florets
- Salt and pepper to taste
- 1 tbsp olive oil

INSTRUCTIONS

1. Toss cut broccoli florets gently with oil.

2. Then season with salt and pepper.
3. Place seasoned broccoli in air fryer basket.
4. Air fry at 150°C for 10 minutes, shaking basket halfway through.
5. Enjoy.

146.   Air Fryer Morel Mushrooms

Total time: 16 minutes
Servings: 4

INGREDIENTS

- 20 morel mushrooms
- 5 oz block of cream cheese
- 3/4 cup crushed cracker mixture

INSTRUCTIONS

1. Wash and de-stem mushrooms.
2. Mix cream cheese and 2 tbsp crushed cracker mixture.
3. Using your fingers, stuffed mushroom with cream cheese mix.
4. Roll gently, Ztuffed mushroom in the remaining crushed cracker mixture.
5. Place coated mushroom in air fryer basket and air fry at 185°C for 5 to 6 minutes.
6. Serve and enjoy.

147.   Air Fryer Stuffed Peppers

Total time: 25 minutes
Servings: 4

INGREDIENTS

- 5 bell peppers, seeds and stem removed
- 15 oz. diced tomatoes
- 1 can kidney beans
- 1/2 cup mozzarella cheese
- 1 tbsp parmesan cheese
- 1 cup cooked rice

INSTRUCTIONS

1. Deseed peppers and scoop substances out.
2. Combine diced tomatoes including the juice, with rice, beans, and flavoring. Spoon into scooped out peppers. Fill nearly to the top.
3. Place in air fryer basket and cook at 180°C for 12 minutes.
4. Top with cheese blend and cook for an additional 3 minutes until cheese has melted.

148. Air Fryer Vegan Cookies

Total time: 25 minutes
Servings: 18

INGREDIENTS

- 1 cup gluten free flour
- 1/4 tsp of baking soda
- 1 tbsp nondairy milk
- 1/2 cup chocolate chips
- 1/4 cup butter
- 1/2 tsp vanilla extract
- 1 tbsp cocoa powder
- 1/3 cup sugar
- Salt

INSTRUCTIONS

1. Mix dry ingredients in a bowl (except chocolate chips).
2. Whisk wet ingredients together to mix.
3. Combine dry and wet ingredients. Fold in chocolate chips.
4. Roll into 1-inch balls and press each ball gently with a fork to flatten.
5. Place in air fryer basket and air fry at 350° C for 7 minutes.

149. Air Fryer Edamame

Total time: 10 minutes
Servings: 4

INGREDIENTS

- 15 oz. Shelled edamame
- 1 tsp olive oil

INSTRUCTIONS

1. In a bowl, toss edamame with oil and place in air fryer basket.
2. Air fry at 195°C for 10 minutes, shaking basket halfway through.
3. Serve and enjoy.

150. Air Fryer Pickles

Total time: 20 minutes
Servings: 2

INGREDIENTS

- 1 jar pickle rounds

- 2 tbsp olive oil
- 1 tsp maple syrup, optional
- 3/4 cup breadcrumbs

INSTRUCTIONS

1. Remove pickles from jar and drain. Then pat dry with paper towels.
2. Add oil to a small bowl and add maple syrup if using.
3. Place breadcrumbs in another bowl.
4. Dip each pickle first in olive oil mixture, then in breadcrumbs. Coat on both sides.
5. Place pickles in air fryer basket without overlapping and air fry at 200°C for 8 minutes, turning halfway through.
6. Serve and enjoy.

151. Air Fryer Jicama Fries

Servings: 2

INGREDIENTS

- 1 jicama, cut into thin strips
- 1 tsp smoked paprika
- 2 tbsp olive oil
- 1/2 tsp garlic powder
- Salt and pepper to taste

INSTRUCTIONS

1. Add jicama fries in a large bowl, garlic powder, smoked paprika, olive oil, salt and pepper.
2. Toss together to combine and coat evenly.
3. Air fry at 200°C for 15 minutes, shaking basket halfway through.
4. Serve with warm ketchup or any dipping sauce of your choice.

152. Spanish Potatoes

Total time: 45 minutes
Servings: 3

INGREDIENTS

- 1 tbsp aquafaba
- 1 1/2 lb. small red potatoes
- 1 tsp tomato paste
- 1/2 tsp brown rice flour
- 1 tsp smoked paprika
- 1 tsp garlic powder
- 1/2 tsp salt

INSTRUCTIONS

1. Boil potatoes. Include 1 tsp of salt if using. Cook for 4 minutes.
2. Add aquafaba and tomato paste in a touch bowl.
3. Blend flour in with the remaining ingredients.
4. Add tomato paste combination to the potatoes and sprinkle the dry seasonings on the potatoes blending tenderly to cover.

153. Vegan Pizza Pockets

Total time: 15 minutes
Servings: 2

INGREDIENTS

- 1 container crescent rolls
- 2 tbsp pasta sauce
- Vegan cheese, shredded
- Cooking spray

INSTRUCTIONS

1. Divide dough into 2 rectangles and seal the cut lines with your fingers.
2. Lay dough down horizontally. Place 2 spoons of sauce into the dough and top with cheese.
3. Seal the pocket shut.

4. Spray air fryer basket and air fry at 200° C for 6 minutes.
5. Flip, spray and cook for another 5 minutes until golden brown.
6. Serve and enjoy.

154. Air Fryer Coated Chickpeas

Total time: 10 minutes
Servings: 2

INGREDIENTS

- 1/4 cup grated parmesan cheese
- 2 tbsp olive oil
- 1 tsp ground black pepper
- 1 can chickpeas, drained and rinsed
- 1 tsp dried oregano
- Salt

INSTRUCTIONS

1. Combine all ingredients in a large bowl and mix chickpeas in until uniformly covered with seasonings.
2. Set air fryer to 200° C and air fry for 5 minutes, shake basket and fry for an additional 5 minutes or until fresh.
3. Serve promptly and enjoy!

5-INGREDIENT AIR FRYER RECIPES

155. Air Fryer Flourless Chocolate Cake

Total time: 2 hours
Servings: 6

INGREDIENTS

- 1 cup cocoa powder
- 4 tbsp raw honey
- 10 eggs
- 10 bananas, ripen
- 1 avocado

INSTRUCTIONS

1. Preheat air fryer to 180°C.
2. Put cocoa powder, eggs, bananas and honey in a blender and blend until very smooth and even.
3. Divide mixture into 3 parts, 2 for cake and 1 for the icing.
4. Pour the 2 parts into 2 cake baking tins and place in air fryer.
5. Air fry at 180° C for 30 to 35 minutes.
6. Remove tins and set aside to cool.
7. To the remaining cake mixture, add avocado until it a much thicker paste is formed.
8. Apply the paste on the top of the first cake and place the second cake on the first to form a sandwich.
9. With the rest of the paste, form an icing around the cake.
10. Place in refrigerator for about an hour.

156. Baked Salmon Fillet Dijon

Total time: 25 minutes
Servings: 6

INGREDIENTS

- 6 oz. fillets salmon
- 4 tbsp Dijon mustard(prepared)
- 1/2 cup breadcrumbs
- 1/2 cup melted butter
- Salt and pepper

INSTRUCTIONS

1. Preheat air fryer to 200°C.
2. Arrange salmon into air fryer basket.

3. Lightly spread mustard over the top of each fillet and season with salt and ground pepper.
4. Add breadcrumbs crumbs to the butter to mix together and spread over fillets.
5. Bake in air fryer for 15 minutes or until crunchy.

157. Baked Zucchini Fries Recipe

INGREDIENTS

- 3 medium zucchinis
- 1/2 cup seasoned bread crumbs
- 2 tbsp grated Parmesan cheese
- 1/4 tsp garlic powder
- 2 large egg white, salt & pepper

INSTRUCTIONS

1. Preheat air fryer to 425 F.
2. In a little bowl, beat egg whites and season with salt and pepper.
3. In another bowl, place breadcrumbs, garlic powder, and cheese and blend well.
4. Plunge zucchini sticks into eggs then into breadcrumbs and cheese blend.
5. Put the breaded zucchini in a single layer in the air fryer and cook for 15-20 minutes.
6. Serve with Ranch or Marinara sauce for dipping.

158. Simple Baked Chicken Breasts

Total time: 40 minutes
Servings: 4

INGREDIENTS

- 4 chicken breast halves, skin removed
- 2 tbsp olive oil
- 1 tbsp salt
- 2 small pinch favorite seasoning
- 1/4 cup water

INSTRUCTIONS

1. Preheat air fryer to 200°C.
2. Apply olive oil on chicken and sprinkle with salt and seasoning. Dredge on both sides.

3. Place chicken in air fryer basket and air fry for 10 minutes.
4. Flip and fry for another 15 minutes.
5. Remove chicken and scrap remains into a bowl.
6. Add in water and drizzle all over your chicken.
7. Enjoy!

159. Breaded Mushrooms

INGREDIENTS

- 250 grams Button mushrooms
- 4g flour and 1 egg
- Breadcrumbs
- 80 grams Finely grated Parmigiano Reggiano cheese
- Salt and pepper

INSTRUCTIONS

1. In a bowl, combine the breadcrumbs in with the Parmigianino cheese and see it to the opposite facet.
2. Pat the mushrooms dry with paper towels.
3. Roll the mushrooms in the flour. Dunk the mushrooms in the egg.
4. Dunk the mushrooms in the breadcrumbs/cheese mix.
5. Cook the Air-Fryer at 180 C for 7 minutes. Shake whilst cooking.

160. Parmesan-Crusted Pork Chops
Total time: 45 minutes
Servings: 4

INGREDIENTS

- 2 eggs
- 2 tsp favorite seasoning
- Nonstick cooking spray
- 4 pork chops, boneless
- 1/2 cup parmesan cheese, grated

INSTRUCTIONS

1. Preheat air fryer to 175°C and spray basket with cooking spray.
2. Mix seasoning and parmesan cheese in a medium bowl.
3. Crack egg and whisk in another bowl.

4. Dip pork chop first into egg, then into seasoning-cheese mixture until evenly coated on both sides.
5. Place in air fryer basket without overlapping and air fry for 40 minutes or until golden brown, flipping halfway through.

161. Air Fryer Zucchini
Servings: 6

INGREDIENTS

- 4 zucchini halves, sliced into strips
- 1 cup breadcrumbs
- 1/2 cup parmesan cheese, grated
- 2 large eggs, whisked
- Cooking spray

INSTRUCTIONS

1. Preheat air fryer to 200°C and spray with non-stick cooking spray.
2. Combine breadcrumbs and cheese in a bowl and mix together.
3. Set whisked eggs aside.
4. Dip zucchini strips first into egg, then into the prepared mixture until evenly coated on both sides.
5. Air fry for 20 to 25 minutes or until golden brown, flipping halfway through cooking.

162. Air fryer Egg Frittata
Total time: 35 minutes
Servings: 2

INGREDIENTS

- 1/2lb cooked sausage, smashed
- 4 eggs, whisked
- ½ cup cheddar cheese, shredded
- 2 red bell pepper, diced
- 1 green onion, chopped.

INSTRUCTIONS

1. Mix eggs, sausage, cheese, onion and bell pepper in a bowl to combine.
2. Preheat air fryer to 180°C and spray air fryer baking pan with cooking spray.
3. Pour egg mixture in baking pan and cook in air fryer for 18 to 20 minutes.
4. When frittata is set, remove and serve!

163. Garlic & Vermouth Roasted Mushrooms

INGREDIENTS

- 1 kg mushrooms
- 1 tbsp duck fat
- 1/2 tsp garlic powder
- 2 tsp herbs de Provence
- 2 tbsp white vermouth

INSTRUCTIONS

1. Wash the mushrooms; turn dry in a plate of mixed greens spinner, quarter them and set aside
2. Put the duck fat, garlic powder, and the herbs de Provence in the air fryer.
3. Warm for 2 minutes. Stir.
4. Add the mushrooms, cook for 25 minutes.
5. Add the white vermouth; cook for an additional 5 minutes.

164. Air Fryer Marinara Pie

INGREDIENTS

- 2- Pizza dough
- 1 chopped tomato
- 1 tbsp olive oil
- 1/2 cloves garlic
- 1/4 tsp sugar
- Salt and basil

INSTRUCTIONS

1. In a skillet, combine all ingredients and cook over medium warm for 45 minutes.
2. Preheat air fryer to 210°C.
3. Roll out mixture and precooked for 4 to 5 minutes.
4. Put a liberal measure of sauce into the pizza mixture.
5. Bake in the air fryer for 18 to 20 minutes. Enjoy!

165. Chickpea & Rosemary Baked Frittata
Servings: 1

INGREDIENTS

- 2 eggs
- 1/4 cup grated parmesan cheese
- 1/2 can chickpeas, drained
- Rosemary leaves, picked
- Seasoning

INSTRUCTIONS

1. Preheat air fryer to 200°C.
2. Spray air fryer baking pan with cooking spray.
3. Whisk eggs and parmesan together and season to taste.
4. Place chickpeas in the air fryer pan, pour in the egg mixture and scatter rosemary on top. Season to taste.
5. Place in the preheated air fryer and air fry for about 15 minutes or until golden and puffy.

166. Air Fryer French Toast Sticks
Total time: 20 minutes
Servings: 4

INGREDIENTS

- 8 slices almost stale bread
- 4 eggs, beaten
- 1/2 cup milk
- 1 tbsp vanilla extract
- 1 tbsp cinnamon

INSTRUCTIONS

1. Preheat air fryer to 180°C.
2. Cut each slice of bread lengthwise.
3. In a bowl, stir together eggs, milk, vanilla extract and cinnamon. Dip each stick of bread into egg mixture, making sure it s evenly coated.
4. Line bottom of air fryer basket with parchment paper.
5. Place bread slices in prepared air fryer basket without overlapping. Air fry for 5 minutes, flip and continue frying for another 5 minutes.

167.   Zucchini Zircles

Total Time: 23minutes

Servings: 3

INGREDIENTS

- 3 large Zucchini and 3/4 cup Milk
- 1/2 cup All-Purpose Flour
- 1 cup Seasoned Dry Italian Breadcrumbs
- 1/2 cup Powdered Sugar

INSTRUCTIONS

1. Line a cookie sheet with paper towels. Wash and dry Zucchini. Cut Zucchini about 1/4 inches thick and put on lined Cookie Sheet.
2. Line up 3 shallow dishes, placing flour in one, milk in the following and Seasoned Breadcrumbs in the third. Coat zucchini in flour, shake off excess and drop into milk. Finally, place Zucchini in a bowl with Breadcrumbs. Coat zucchini and put onto wire baking rack.
3. In a single layer, delicately place zucchini in air fryer basket and utilize an oil mister to grease well with oil.
4. Cook at 390 F for 8 minutes, cautiously flipping one-part of the way through.
5. Remove from Air Fryer and sprinkle with Powdered Sugar.

168.   Air Fryer Chicken Quesadilla

Total time: 15 minutes

Servings: 2

INGREDIENTS

- 2 flour tortillas
- 1/2 chicken breast, chopped
- 1/4 cup cooked onions
- 1/2 cup cooked peppers-green and red
- 1/2 cup parmesan cheese

INSTRUCTIONS

1. Preheat air fryer to 200°C.
2. Line air fryer skillet with wax paper.
3. Place 1 flour tortilla on a working table and top with chicken, pepper, onion, and cheese.
4. Place another tortilla on top and press softly.
5. Transfer to air fryer and cook for 10 minutes until cheese has completely softened.

169.   Roasted Parmesan Rosemary Potatoes

Total time: 55 minutes

Servings: 4

INGREDIENTS

- 2 pounds potatoes cut into pieces
- 1 tbsp chopped rosemary (fresh)
- 3 tbsp extra virgin olive oil
- 2 tbsp parmesan cheese (grated)

INSTRUCTIONS

1. Preheat air fryer to 220 C and line basket with aluminum foil.
2. Place potatoes in a bowl and add parmesan cheese, olive oil and rosemary, mixing them together. Season with salt and pepper or to taste.
3. Place potatoes and spread in a single layer over air fryer basket.
4. Bake for about 40 minutes, until potatoes are golden brown and tender.
5. Turn once halfway through baking.

170.   Baked Italian Chicken

Total time: 1-hour

Servings: 4

INGREDIENTS

- Cooking spray
- 1-pound skinless, boneless chicken breast, diced.
- 10 oz. broccoli
- 4 potatoes, diced
- 7 oz. Italian dressing mix and quarter butter.

INSTRUCTIONS

1. Preheat air fryer to 175 C.
2. Spray basket evenly with cooking spray.
3. Spread chicken, broccoli, potatoes into basket and sprinkle with Italian dressing.
4. Bake for 45 to 55 minutes. & it's ready!

171.   Simple Soba Noodle Soup

Total Time: 10 minutes

Servings: 1

INGREDIENTS

- 2 cups vegetable stock.
- 50 grams of soba noodles.
- 3 heads baby bok choy (leaves separated) or baby spinach.
- 1/4 tbsp chili flakes
- 1 1/2 tbsp soy sauce

INSTRUCTIONS

1. Pour stock into a medium cooking bowl and place in air fryer.
2. Boil, add noodles and simmer for 2 minutes.
3. Add bok choy, chili and soy sauce to broth and simmer for one more minute (noodles can be slightly undercooked)
4. Remove from air fryer. Taste and serve hot.

172.   Air Fryer Boxty Pancakes

Total time: 15 minutes

Servings: 3

INGREDIENTS

- 1/2 cup mashed potatoes
- 1 small potato, shredded
- 1/4 cup buttermilk
- 1/2 cup all-purpose flour
- Salt and pepper to taste

INSTRUCTIONS

1. Place mashed potatoes in a large bowl.
2. Grate raw potato into a mesh sieve.
3. Sprinkle salt on raw potato and press into the sieve to remove excess water.
4. Combine mashed potatoes, raw potato, buttermilk, flour and pepper and salt in a large bowl.
5. Line air fryer baking pan with parchment paper and cut out desired amount of boxty into the pan.
6. Spray with generous amount of cooking spray and transfer to air fryer.
7. Bake 4 to 5 minutes, flip and bake for another 5 minutes at 160°C or until golden brown.
8. Serve and enjoy!

173.   Air Fryer Carrot Cake

Total Time: 45 minutes

Serving: 6

INGREDIENTS

- 1/2 cup brown sugar
- 1/2 cup melted butter
- 2 eggs
- All-purpose flour.
- 3 cups carrots, shredded

INSTRUCTIONS

1. In a medium bowl, combine sugar and butter.
2. Add eggs and blend completely for even mix. Mix in flour and carrots.
3. Pour cake batter into greased cake tin.
4. Place the cupcake tins into the air fryer container without covering.
5. Air fry at 175°C until fork embedded into the inside tells the truth.
6. Allow cake to cool and top with your preferred icing.

174.   Air Fryer Zucchini Chips

Total time: 20 minutes

Servings: 4

INGREDIENTS

- 2 zucchinis, sliced thinly
- 2 eggs, paprika
- 1/2 cup breadcrumbs
- 5 tbsp flour
- Cooking spray

INSTRUCTIONS

1. Whisk egg in a small bowl.
2. Combine crumbs, flour and paprika in another small bowl.
3. Dip each zucchini slice into egg and then in the crumb mixture. Be sure it sticks.
4. Place zucchini slices into the air fryer in a single layer, spray lightly with cooking spray, and cook at 200 C for 8 to 10 minutes.
5. Flip at intervals. Enjoy with any dipping sauce of your choice.

175. Air Fryer French Fries

Total time: 1hr 20minutes
Servings: 1

INGREDIENTS

- 1 russet potato
- 1/2 tsp garlic salt
- Cooking spray
- 1/4 tsp onion powder

INSTRUCTIONS

1. Preheat air fryer to 380 F
2. Soak potatoes in a medium bowl containing water for around 60 minutes.
3. Drain water and toss fries with onion powder and garlic salt.
4. Place fries in the air fryer crate without covering. Grease with cooking oil and cook for 20 minutes. Turn partially through. Serve.

176. Shoestring Carrots

Total Time: 18 minutes
Serving: 3

INGREDIENTS

- 10- oz. of julienned carrots
- 1 tbsp olive oil
- salt and pepper
- apple cider vinegar in a spray bottle
- 1 tsp orange zest

INSTRUCTIONS

1. In a medium bowl, blend the carrots in with the olive oil, covering them softly.
2. Season with salt and pepper.
3. Put the carrots florets in an air fryer set at 390 F. Cook for 13 minutes, shaking at regular intervals.
4. Move them to a serving bowl, mix with orange zest, splash a little apple juice vinegar, and salt and pepper.
5. Serve immediately.

177. Air Fryer Sweet Potato Fries

Total time: 15minutes
Servings: 4

INGREDIENTS

- 2 large sweet potatoes
- 1 tbsp red pepper flakes
- 1 tbsp olive oil
- Salt to taste
- Pepper

INSTRUCTIONS

1. Preheat air fryer to 180 C.
2. Coat sweet potatoes with olive oil in a medium bowl.
3. Toss red pepper flakes, pepper, and salt into potatoes until completely blanketed.
4. Transfer potatoes to preheated air fryer and cook for 10 minutes.
5. Toss for the duration of cooking.

178. Air Fryer Crusted Salmon

Total time: 12 minutes
Servings: 4

INGREDIENTS

- 10 oz. salmon filets
- 8 fresh mint leaves, chopped
- 1/2 cup salad cream
- Seasoning
- Lemon juice

INSTRUCTIONS

1. Preheat air fryer to 200C.
2. Season salmon with seasoning to taste.
3. Mix cream with mint and lemon juice in a bowl and apply medium amount over each salmon.
4. Spray lightly with cooking spray and fry for 6 minutes or until cooked properly.

179. Crispy Air Fryer Chicken Wings

Total Time: 25 minutes
Servings: 4

INGREDIENTS

- 1 1/2 lbs. chicken wings
- kosher salt
- black pepper
- garlic powder
- Cooking spray

INSTRUCTIONS

1. Preheat air fryer to 200 C.
2. Season wings to taste with salt, dark pepper, and garlic powder.
3. Place prepared wings in the air fryer basket without covering.
4. Cook the wings in air fryer for 12 to 15 minutes, flip and resume cooking for another 10-15 minutes.

180. Air Fryer Loaded Potatoes

Total time: 25 minutes
Servings: 2

INGREDIENTS

- 8 baby Yukon gold potatoes
- 1 tsp olive oil
- 1 1/2 tbsp chopped chives
- 1/8 tsp kosher salt
- 2 bacon slices, 2 tbsp reduced fat cream/ cheddar.

INSTRUCTIONS

1. Coat potatoes with oil and place in air fryer basket to cook for 25 minutes at 350 F, until fork tender.
2. Stir occasionally.
3. Still at the same time, cook bacon in pan over medium heat for 7 minutes until crispy.
4. Remove and crumble with your hand.
5. Place potatoes on a flat plate and crush lightly till it splits open.
6. Top with crumbled bacon, drippings, chives, sour cream, cheese and salt.
7. Serve.

181. Air Fryer Roasted Broccoli

Total time: 20 minutes
Servings: 4

INGREDIENTS

- 12 oz. Broccoli
- 10 tbsp evaporated milk, low in fat
- Cooking spray
- 5 tbsp fresh Mexican cheese
- 6 saltine crackers, 3 tbsp Amarillo paste.

INSTRUCTIONS

1. Spray broccoli florets with cooking spray and place in air fryer basket without overlapping.
2. Cook at 375°F for 7 minutes until crispy and tender.
3. Blend evaporated milk, cheese, paste and saltines together until smooth.
4. Pour mixture into a bowl and microwave for about 30 seconds.
5. Serve sauce with broccoli.

182. Air Fryer Toad-In-The-Hole Tarts

Total time: 30 minutes
Servings: 4

INGREDIENTS

- 4 tbsp cheddar, shredded.
- 4 tbsp cooked ham, diced
- 4 eggs
- 1 sheet puff pastry, thawed
- Chives, fresh and chopped

INSTRUCTIONS

1. Preheat air fryer to 200°C
2. Cut pastry sheets into 4 squares
3. Place first 2 pastries into air fryer basket and cook for 7 minutes
4. Remove air fryer basket and press each pastry with a spoon to make a hole. Into the hole created, place 1 tbsp cheese and ham and Pour one egg on top.
5. Return basket to air fryer, cook for another 5 minutes.
6. Remove and repeat for remaining 2 pastry squares.

183. Air Fryer Scrambled Egg Muffin

Total time: 30 minutes
Servings: 6

INGREDIENTS

- 6 eggs
- 1/2-pound pork sausage
- 1/2 cup chopped green pepper and onion
- 1/2 cup cheddar cheese, shredded
- 1/2 tbsp salt and garlic powder

INSTRUCTIONS

1. Preheat air fryer to 175° F.

2. Lightly oil 6 biscuit tins
3. Add wiener to a saucer over medium-high warm.
4. Cook and mix for 10 to 15 minutes or until frankfurter are equally dark-colored and brittle.
5. Beat eggs into a bowl. Include onion, green pepper, garlic powder, and salt and mix.
6. Include cooked hotdog and cheese and blend.
7. Fill into arranged biscuit tins.
8. Place biscuit tins into the air fryer group by clump and heat for 22 to 25 minutes or until fork embedded into the middle confesses all.
9. Repeat for the residual bunch.
10. Serve hot for breakfast!

184.   Air Fryer Kale Chips
Total time: 28 minutes
Servings: 2

INGREDIENTS

- 6 cups packed kale leaves, de-stemmed.
- 1 tbsp extra-virgin olive oil
- 1 tsp soy sauce, low in sodium
- 1 tsp black sesame seeds
- 1/2 tsp dried garlic, minced
- Poppy seeds (optional)

INSTRUCTIONS

1. Wash and dry kale leaves and attack pieces.
2. Toss with olive oil and soy sauce in a bowl ensuring the leaves are covered equitably.
3. Place piece of kale leaves in air fryer basket and cook at 188°C for 6 minutes or until fresh.
4. Shake basket partially through cooking.
5. Place kale leaves on a level sheet and sprinkles with sesame seeds, poppy seeds, and garlic.
6. Repeat for the residual group. Serve nibble.
7. minutes or until fork embedded into the middle confesses all.
8. Repeat for the outstanding cluster.
9. Serve hot for breakfast!

185.   Air-fryer Ricotta Balls
Total time: 20 minutes
Servings: 20

INGREDIENTS

- 250g ricotta

- 15g chopped basil, fresh
- 1 egg
- 2 tbsp flour
- 3 slices stale bread pepper, freshly ground.
- 1 tbsp chives, chopped

INSTRUCTIONS

1. Preheat air fryer to 200°C
2. Combine ricotta, flour and egg yolk in a bowl and mix properly.
3. Add salt and pepper. Add chives and basil.
4. Mold mixture into 20 little balls. Leave balls to rest.
5. Prepare breadcrumbs in a large bowl.
6. Beat egg white into another.
7. Coat each ball with egg white in a bowl and toss with breadcrumbs.
8. Place balls in air fryer basket without overlapping and cook for 8 to 10 minutes

186.   Mac & Cheese
Total time: 40 minutes
Servings: 2

INGREDIENTS

- 2 cups dry macaroni
- 1 tsp cornstarch
- 2 cups shredded Cheddar
- 2 cups whipped cream
- Salt, optional

INSTRUCTIONS

1. Mix half cup cheese and cornstarch with other ingredients.
2. Scoop mixture into the baking dish of air fryer and place aluminum foil over it.
3. Cook for 15 minutes at 310° F, remove foil after 15 minutes and add remaining cheese.
4. Cook for another 10 minutes.

187.   Ricotta and Spinach Filo Pastry
Total time: 10 minutes
Servings: 4

INGREDIENTS

- 500g baby spinach
- 1 egg
- 250g ricotta cheese

- 4 sheets filo pastry
- 30g pine nuts and/or 1 lemon zest

INSTRUCTIONS

1. Steam spinach in microwave or boiling water for 30 seconds. Drain.
2. Chop drained spinach and combine with ricotta, lemon zest, egg and nuts.
3. Season to taste.
4. Divide filo sheets into 3 triangular strips.
5. Add 1 tbsp of mixture into the large end of each strip.
6. Fold into a triangle and place in air fryer.
7. Fry at 200° C for 4 minutes.

188.   Mozzarella Cheese Sticks

Total time: 30 minutes
Servings: 8

INGREDIENTS

- 16 oz. mozzarella cheese block, sliced into 1/4-inch stick
- 3 tbsp low-fat milk
- 2 eggs, beaten
- 1 cup breadcrumbs, Italian flavored
- 1/4 cup plain flour

INSTRUCTIONS

1. Mix egg and milk in a little bowl.
2. Prepare breadcrumbs and flour in a medium bowl.
3. Dip cheese sticks into flour then into egg blend and into breadcrumb.
4. Ensure each stick is uniformly covered.
5. Place sticks in air fryer and fry for 10 minutes at 200°C.

189.   Air Fryer Honey Barbeque Chicken Wings

Total time: 35 minutes
Servings: 10

INGREDIENTS

- 10 chicken wings
- 1/2 cup flour
- 1/2 BBQ sauce
- Kosher salt and chili powder
- 1/4 cup honey

INSTRUCTIONS

1. Preheat air fryer to 180°C
2. In a large bowl, combine flour, chili powder, salt, paprika.
3. Dunk wings in blend and coat uniformly
4. Place chicken wings in the air fryer bin without covering and cook for 15 minutes, flipping part of the way through, until fresh.
5. Combine honey and BBQ sauce n another bowl and coat bubbled wings with a cooking brush.
6. Cook again at 180°C for another 8 to 10 minutes or until sauce is caramelized.
7. Serve and enjoy it!

190.   Air Fryer Dry-Rubbed Chicken Wings

Total time: 30 minutes
Servings: 12

INGREDIENTS

- 12 chicken wings
- 1 tsp garlic powder
- 1 tsp chili powder
- 1/2 tsp kosher salt
- 1/2 black pepper, paprika

INSTRUCTIONS

1. Preheat air fryer to 180°C
2. Mix garlic powder, chili powder, paprika, salt and pepper in a large bowl.
3. Rinse and pat every chicken wing dry and toss into a bowl to cover uniformly.
4. Place wings in air fryer crate and cook for 15 minutes, turning at interims.
5. Cool again for an additional 5 minutes.
6. Serve hot.

191.   Air Fryer Marinated Chicken Wings

Total time: 1hour 20minutes
Servings: 12

INGREDIENTS

- 12 chicken wings, thawed
- 1/2 cup olive oil
- 1 tsp chili powder
- 1 tsp paprika
- 1 tsp salt

INSTRUCTIONS

1. Preheat air fryer to 200°C.
2. Join olive oil, paprika, salt and chili in a large bowl.
3. Dip chicken wings in blend and marinate for 45 minutes.
4. Place marinated wings into air fryer basket and fry for 12 minutes.
5. Shake basket. Cook for an additional 8 minutes.
6. Remove and serve.

192.   Air Fryer Spinach Pakora

Total time: 30minutes
Servings: 4

INGREDIENTS

- 4 large handfuls spinach, chopped
- 1 Onion, chopped, 1 green chilies, chopped
- 3 small ginger, chopped
- 1/2 tbsp chickpea and rice flour
- 1/2 curry powder and salt
- Water

INSTRUCTIONS

1. Place spinach, onions, green chilies and ginger in a bowl, and include salt and chili powder.
2. Add chickpea flour and rice flour and mix well. Include 1/2 cup water.
3. Spray Air fryer container with cooking oil and scoop the batter blend into the basket, without covering.
4. Cook at 185°C for 6 to 7 minutes. Flip and press delicately with the back of a spoon. Cook for an additional 8 minutes and serve.

193.   Air Fryer Tortellini Pasta Salad

Total time: 30 minutes
Servings: 2

INGREDIENTS

- 1 pack cheese tortellini, freshly refrigerated
- 1 cucumber, finely chopped
- 2 finely chopped red bell peppers
- 1/2 cup Italian salad dressing
- 1/2 cup Parmesan cheese, shredded

INSTRUCTIONS

1. Cook pasta in air fryer prospect minutes at 150°C. Let cool.
2. In a large bowl, combine pasta, cucumber, bell pepper, a serving of mixed greens dressing and cheese, and blend well.
3. Refrigerate for 2 hours or more.

194.   Air Fryer Crispy Chicken Dinner Recipe

Total time: 18 minutes
Servings: 4

INGREDIENTS

- 2 chicken breasts.
- 1/2 cup breadcrumbs
- 1 cup low fat milk
- 1 cup shaved Parmesan cheese, shredded
- salt and pepper to taste

INSTRUCTIONS

1. Preheat air fryer to 200°C. Spray cooking basket lightly with cooking spray.
2. Place milk and chicken breasts in a large bowl. Add a large pinch of salt and ground pepper.
3. Marinate for 10 minutes.
4. In another bowl, mix breadcrumbs and shredded cheese.
5. Put mixture on top of chicken breast by pressing it, making sure it's well coasted. Place in air fryer basket. Spray chicken lightly with cooking spray.
6. Cook in preheated air fryer for 8 minutes, flipping halfway through.

195.   Air Fryer Empanadas

Total time: 18 minutes
Servings: 5

INGREDIENTS

- 1 pie crust, refrigerated
- 3 slices deli Swiss cheese, chopped into small pieces
- 1/4-pound deli ham, thinly sliced and cut into small pieces
- 3 small dill pickles, cut into small pieces
- 1 1/2 tbsp mustard

INSTRUCTIONS

1. Preheat air fryer to 175°C.
2. Cut 10 circles out of pie crust, and spread mustard onto each.
3. Add a slice of ham, cheese, and pickles.
4. Crease the empty end over to cover the fillings and pleat edges together with a fork.
5. Grease air fryer container with cooking oil, place empanadas batters into the bin and splash again with cooking oil.
6. Cook for 8 minutes, flipping part way through. Remove from air fryer and enjoy!

196. Air Fryer Lemon Chicken

Total time: 25 minutes
Servings: 2

INGREDIENTS

- 6 chicken tenderloins
- 2 eggs
- 1 1/2 cups breadcrumbs
- Kosher salt
- 2 lemons, halved

INSTRUCTIONS

1. Beat 2 eggs into a small bowl. In another large bowl, empty breadcrumbs.
2. Dip each chicken in egg, coating on both sides. Dredge both sides in breadcrumbs.
3. Set air fryer to 200°C and place coated chicken in air fryer basket.
4. Cook for 14 to 15 minutes, flipping halfway through.
5. Transfer cooked chicken into a baking dish lined with paper towels and sprinkle with some salt.
6. Squeeze lemon juice on top.

197. Air Fryer Beef Roast

Total time: 40 minutes + 5 hours to marinate
Servings: 4

INGREDIENTS

- 3-pound beef chuck, thawed
- 3 tbsp soy sauce
- 1/2 cup orange juice
- 3 tbsp brown sugar
- 1 tsp salt, pepper

INSTRUCTIONS

1. Combine orange juice, soy sauce and darker sugar in a bowl. Mix well.
2. Pour blend over hamburger meat and marinate for 4 to 5 hours.
3. Place marinated meat in the air fryer bin and sprinkle with salt and pepper.
4. Cook for 30 minutes at 200°C, flipping part of the way through.

198. Air Fryer Easy Burger

Total time: 20 minutes
Servings: 4

INGREDIENTS

- 4 ground beef
- 1 1/2 tsp Worcestershire Sauce
- 1 tsp salt
- 1/2 tsp pepper
- 1/2 tsp garlic powder

INSTRUCTIONS

1. In a large bowl, combine sauce, pepper, and salt and garlic powder.
2. Divide blend and put into 4 even patties. Press to pack.
3. Spray air fryer basket with cooking oil and place every patty in.
4. Set Air fry to 200°C and fry for 6 minutes.
5. Flip and keep searching for an additional 4 minutes.
6. Add your preferred ingredients and enjoy it!

199. Air Fryer Corn on the Cob

Total time: 10 minutes
Servings: 3

INGREDIENTS

- 3 ears fresh corn, de-husked and trimmed
- Cooking spray
- Salt
- Pepper
- Butter

INSTRUCTIONS

1. Preheat air fryer to 200°C.
2. Spray corn with cooking spray.
3. Season to taste with salt and pepper.

4. Place in air fryer basket without overlapping.
5. Cook for 10 minutes, flipping halfway through. Butter corn and enjoy!

200. Air Fryer Baked Potatoes
Total time: 45 minutes
Servings: 4

INGREDIENTS

- 4 large potatoes
- 2 tbsp olive oil
- Kosher salt and pepper
- Garlic powder
- 4 tbsp butter
- Parsley, optional

INSTRUCTIONS

1. Rub the skin of potatoes with olive oil.
2. Sprinkle with salt, pepper, garlic powder and parsley.
3. Place in air fryer basket and cook for 45 minutes at 200°C.
4. When done, cut potatoes delicately and mash with butter.

201. Air Fryer Easy Coated Shrimp
Total time: 30 minutes
Servings: 4

INGREDIENTS

- 12 cooked shrimp
- 1/2 tsp black pepper and garlic powder
- 1/2 cup all-purpose flour and paprika
- 2 eggs, beaten
- 1 cup Breadcrumbs

INSTRUCTIONS

1. Combine pepper and garlic powder in a small bowl and sprinkle generously over shrimp.
2. In another bowl, combine flour and paprika.
3. Whisk eggs in one bowl and place breadcrumbs in another.
4. Dip both sides of each shrimp into flour mixture, then into egg and finally coat with breadcrumbs.
5. Place coated shrimps in sprayed air fryer basket.
6. Spray again with nonstick cooking spray.

7. Then fry at 175°C for 10 minutes, when crumbs turn golden.
8. Serve with any dipping sauce of your choice.

202. Air Fryer Easy Pizza
Total time: 25 minutes
Servings: 4

INGREDIENTS

- Pre-made 10" pizza crust
- Pizza sauce
- Tomatoes, sliced
- Mozzarella cheese, shredded and cubed
- Onions or any topping of your choice

INSTRUCTIONS

1. Preheat air fryer to 175°C
2. Drizzle pizza sauce generously over the pizza crust
3. Add shredded cheese, tomato slices and onions.
4. Sprinkle mozzarella cheese cube all over pizza.
5. Bake in preheated air fryer for 10 minutes or until cheese is bubbly.
6. Slice and enjoy!

203. Air Fryer Easy Cake
Total time: 30 minutes
Servings: 4

INGREDIENTS

- 6 tbsp sugar
- 2 eggs
- 1/4 cup flour
- 1/4 tsp of baking soda
- 1/2 tsp cream of tartar
- Flavor, vanilla

INSTRUCTIONS

1. Beat eggs and add sugar. Mix on high for 7 minutes.
2. Add vanilla flavor, flour, baking soda and cream of tartar and mix on medium for 1 minute.
3. Empty batter into already greased air fryer cake pan.
4. Bake at 165°C for 15 minutes or until cake is golden brown

5. Cool and serve with any toppings of your choice such as whipped cream and chocolate chips.
6. Enjoy!

204. **Air Fryer Glazed Donuts**

Total time: 12 minutes

Servings: 4

INGREDIENTS

- Grands! Biscuits, 4 pieces
- 1/4 cup chocolate cream
- 1 cup powdered sugar
- 2 tbsp milk
- Toppings of your choice

INSTRUCTIONS

1. Cut out the center of every scone utilizing a doughnut shaper.
2. Grease air fryer bin with cooking oil and place 4 doughnuts in it.
3. Air fry at 165°C for 4 to 5 minutes. Remove and allow to cool.
4. In a large bowl, mix sugar, chocolate cream until smooth.
5. Dip one side of each doughnut into cream.

205.   Air Fryer Breakfast Omelet

Total time: 20 minutes
Servings: 1

INGREDIENTS

- 2 large eggs
- 1/4 cup low-fat milk
- 1/4 tsp salt
- Fresh meat and vegetables of your choice (green onions, red bell pepper, ham)
- 1 tsp herb seasoning

INSTRUCTIONS

1. Combine eggs and milk in a bowl until well blended.
2. Add salt and veggies to egg mixture.
3. Grease air fryer pan and pour mixture into it.
4. Place pan into the air fryer basket and cook at 175°C for 8-10 minutes.
5. Sprinkle herb seasoning on omelet halfway through cooking.

206.   Air Fryer Crispy Avocado Wedges

Total time: 15 to 20 minutes
Servings: 2

INGREDIENTS

- 1 tbsp garlic pepper
- 1/2 cup all-purpose flour
- 2 eggs, beaten
- 1 cup Breadcrumbs
- 2 avocados, cut into 4 wedges each

INSTRUCTIONS

1. Mix flour and garlic pepper in a large bowl or container.
2. Add eggs to another bowl.

3. Place Breadcrumb pieces in the third bowl.
4. Coat avocado wedges in flour blend, eggs, then breadcrumbs.
5. Spray air fryer crate with a cooking oil and place avocado wedges in it. Splash once more.
6. Cook at 200°C for 8 minutes, turning partway through.

207.   Air Fryer Pork Taquitos

Total time: 25 minutes
Servings: 10

INGREDIENTS

- 3 cups pork tenderloin, cooked and shredded
- 3 cups low-fat mozzarella cheese, shredded
- 10 small flour or corn tortillas
- 2 tbsp lime juice, squeezed
- Non-stick cooking spray

INSTRUCTIONS

1. Preheat air fryer to 190°C
2. Drizzle lime juice over pork.
3. Place 4 oz. meat and 1/4 cup cheese into each tortilla.
4. Roll tortillas into taquitos.
5. Use a toothpick to hold taquito along the seam and place each in greased air fryer bin.
6. Spray liberally with cooking oil.
7. Fry for 8 to 10 minutes, flipping halfway through.

208.   Air Fryer Chicken Taquitos

Total time: 26 minutes
Servings: 12

INGREDIENTS

- 4 cups salsa chicken or chicken tenderloin (cooked and diced)
- 12 tbsp mozzarella cheese, shredded
- 12 small flour or corn tortillas
- Cooking spray

INSTRUCTIONS

1. Preheat air fryer to 200°C.
2. Place 2 tbsp shredded chicken and 1 tbsp shredded cheese into one end of each tortilla.
3. Roll carefully from filled end to form taquito.
4. Use a toothpick to hold taquito along the seam

5. Spray air fryer basket with cooking spray and place taquitos into the basket without overlapping.
6. Spray again.
7. Air fry for 6 to 7 minutes or until taquito is golden brown.

209.   Air Fryer Tortilla Chips
Total time: 14 minutes
Servings: 1+

INGREDIENTS

- Flour or corn tortillas
- Pepper, optional
- Salt to taste
- Cooking spray
- Dipping sauce, optional

INSTRUCTIONS

1. Preheat air fryer to 175°C
2. Using a cookie cutter, cut each tortilla in circles.
3. Spray the 2 sides of every tortilla round with cooking oil.
4. Sprinkle the 2 sides with salt and pepper.
5. Spray air fryer basket with a cooking oil, at that point place around 9 to 10 rounds into the bin.
6. Air fry for 2 to 3 minutes, flip and proceed for another 2 to 3 minutes.

210.   Air Fryer Mini Apple Pies
Total time: 20 minutes
Servings: 4

INGREDIENTS

- 4 oz. 9" pie crust
- 4 tbsp blended apple (for apple pie filling)
- 4 caramel squares
- Coarse sugar
- Cooking spray

INSTRUCTIONS

1. Preheat air fryer to 175°C.
2. Unroll pie covering. Utilizing a 4.5-inch round shaper, cut out 4 rounds.
3. Fill each round with 1 tbsp apple and place 1 caramel square on the filling.
4. Moisten the edges of each round with water.

5. Using a fork, tenderly press creases together firmly.
6. Make 3-light cuts over every pie. Splash with cooking oil and coarse sugar.
7. Spray air fryer container with cooking oil and place pies in the bin, 2 at once.
8. Air fry for 11 minutes.

211.   Air Fryer Chicken Tenders
Total: 18 minutes
Servings: 4

INGREDIENTS

- 1-pound chicken tenders, uncooked
- 2 tbsp buttermilk
- 1/4 cup Honey
- 1/2 cups breadcrumbs
- 1/2 cup walnuts, crushed or grated
- Salt

INSTRUCTIONS

1. Place raw chicken in a large bowl.
2. Add honey and buttermilk and mix to blend. Give it a chance to rest for around 30 minutes.
3. Place pecans, salt and breadcrumb morsels in a Ziploc pack and shake to combine.
4. Place chicken fingers into the pack, seal and shake together until it is all around covered on all sides.
5. Preheat air fryer to 200°C and grease air fryer bin with cooking oil.
6. Place chicken fingers in the air fryer bin and air fry for 8 minutes.

212.   Air Fryer Crispy Tofu
Total time: 55 minutes
Servings: 4

INGREDIENTS

- 1 firm tofu
- 2 tbsp soy sauce
- 2 tbsp sesame oil
- 1 tbsp cornstarch
- 1 tsp rice vinegar

INSTRUCTIONS

1. Toss tofu, soy sauce, sesame oil and vinegar in a bowl.

2. Marinate for 20 to 30 minutes.
3. Sprinkle marinated tofu liberally with cornstarch.
4. Place tofu into air fryer crate and cook at 185°C for 20 minutes.
5. Shake container part of the way through.

213. Buffalo Cauliflower

Total time: 20 minutes
Servings: 4

INGREDIENTS

- 4 cups cauliflower florets
- 1 cup breadcrumbs combined with coarse salt
- 1/4 cup butter, melted
- 1/4 cup buffalo sauce
- Any creamy salad dressing of your choice

INSTRUCTIONS

1. Whisk buffalo sauce into dissolved butter.
2. Hold every floret by the stem and plunge into the spread blend.
3. Dredge covered florets in the scrap blend, covering it liberally.
4. Place in the air fryer bin and cook at 175°C for 15 to 18 minutes, shaking a couple of times.

214. Air Fryer Breadcrumb Tofu

Total time: 1hour 30minutes
Servings: 4

INGREDIENTS

- 1 block firm tofu
- 1/4 cup soy sauce
- 1 cup breadcrumb bread
- 1/2 cup mayonnaise, vegan
- Ginger-garlic powder

INSTRUCTIONS

1. Place tofu cutlets on a plate and pour mixture over it. Leave to marinate for around 30 to 50 minutes.
2. Pour breadcrumb-salt combo into a bowl. Empty some mayo into another bowl.
3. Dredge tofu cutlets in mayo, then in breadcrumbs.

4. Place tofu cutlets in air fryer without overlapping and cook at 185°C for 20 minutes, shaking bin after 10 minutes.

215. Air Fryer Seasoned Chickpeas

Total time: 25 minutes
Servings: 4

INGREDIENTS

- 1 can chickpeas, drained
- 2 tbsp lemon juice
- 2 tbsp olive oil
- 1 tsp coarse salt
- 1 batch ranch seasoning

INSTRUCTIONS

1. In a bowl, toss together chickpeas and 1 tbsp olive oil.
2. Pour chickpeas in air fryer basket and air fry at 200°C for 15 minutes.
3. Remove and transfer chickpeas back to the bowl.
4. Toss with remaining olive oil, lemon juice, ranch seasoning and salt.
5. Transfer chickpeas back in air fryer basket and cook for another 5 minutes.
6. Serve and enjoy!

216. Air Fryer French Toast Sticks

Total time: 15 minutes
Servings: 2

INGREDIENTS

- 4 slices of bread
- 2 tbsp soft butter
- 2 eggs, lightly beaten
- 1 pinch cinnamon
- 1 pinch ground cloves
- Salt

INSTRUCTIONS

1. Preheat air fryer to 180°C.
2. In a bowl, mix beaten eggs, a sprinkle of salt, a touch of cinnamon, and ground cloves.
3. Generously apply spread to both sides of bread cuts and cut them into strips.
4. Dip each piece of bread in egg blend. Place in the air fryer bin in a single layer.

5. Cook for 2 minutes. Spray bread with cooking oil.
6. Return container to air fryer and cook for an additional 4 minutes.

217.   Air Fryer Breakfast Bomb

Total time: 30 minutes
Servings: 4

INGREDIENTS

- 3 bacon slices
- 3 eggs, lightly beaten
- 1 oz cream cheese, softened
- 1 tbsp fresh chives, chopped
- 4 oz. fresh whole-wheat pizza dough
- Cooking spray

INSTRUCTIONS

1. Place bacon in a sauce skillet and cook over medium heat for around 10 minutes or until fresh.
2. Remove bacon, place in a sha low bowl, and crumble.
3. Add beaten eggs to bacon in skillet and cook for 4 minutes.
4. Transfer cooked eggs to a bowl, and add the cream cheese, crumbled bacon and chives.
5. Cut pizza dough into 4 equal parts.
6. Fold each segment into a 5-inch circle and place one segment of egg blend in each.
7. Brush edge of the mixture with water, fold dough over filling and squeeze the creases firmly.
8. Place mixture in air fryer container, grease with cooking oil. Air fry at 175°C for 6 minutes.

218.   Air Fryer Cheese and Veggie Egg Cups

Total time: 30 minutes
Servings: 4

INGREDIENTS

- 4 large eggs, whisked
- 1 cup veggies of choice, diced
- 1 cup cheese, shredded
- 1 tbsp cilantro, chopped
- 4 tbsp half-and-half cream
- Salt and Pepper

INSTRUCTIONS

1. In a bowl, whisk eggs, vegetables, 1/2 cup cheese, cilantro, cream, salt and pepper.
2. Divide and place into 4 greased ramekins or baking cup.
3. Place ramekins in air fryer basket, set the temperature to 150°C and cook for 12 minutes.
4. After 12 minutes, add remaining cheese on top.
5. Set air fryer to 200° C and cook for another 2 minutes until cheese has melted.

219.   Air Fryer Crab Rangoon

Total time: 40 minutes
Servings: 10

INGREDIENTS

- 1/2-pound chive and onion cream cheese
- 1 can crab meat
- 30 wonton wrapper doughs
- 3 tbsp olive oil
- Cooking spray

INSTRUCTIONS

1. Combine crab meat and cream cheese in a medium bowl
2. Place wonton wrappers on a flat surface and place 1 tbsp of filling in the center of the wrapper. Brush the edges of the wrappers with water to assist seal.
3. Fold over and delicately press creases collectively. Brush with olive oil.
4. Place wontons in air fryer basket in a single layer and cook at 165°C for 6-8 minutes

220.   Air Fryer Meatballs

Total time: 30 minutes
Servings: 6

INGREDIENTS

- 1 lb. lean ground beef
- 1 egg
- onions
- 1/2 cup breadcrumbs
- 1/2 cup ketchup
- 1/2 tbsp hot sauce
- Salt and pepper

INSTRUCTIONS

1. Chop onions into little pieces
2. In a large bowl, combine all ingredients with the ground meat and mix it with your hands.
3. Shape blend into 24 balls.
4. Place 12 meatballs at a time into the air fryer bin and cook at 190°C for 15 minutes.

221. Air Fryer Easy Chocolate Brownies

Total time: 30-35 minutes
Servings: 15

INGREDIENTS

- 1 pack brownie mix
- 3 tbsp olive oil
- 1 large egg
- Water
- Whipped cream topping, optional

INSTRUCTIONS

1. Pour brownie mix in a large bowl and add water, oil and egg.
2. Mix properly for 5 minutes to achieve an even blend.
3. Grease air fryer pan and pour in mixture.
4. Bring to a consistent level with a spatula.
5. Place pan into the air fryer and cook at 160°C for 20 to 25 minutes or until you stick a knife into the brownie and it comes out clean.

222. Air Fryer Fried Shrimp

Total time: 25 minutes
Servings: 4

INGREDIENTS

- 1-pound raw shrimp, peeled
- 1/2 cup all-purpose flour
- 1 cup breadcrumbs
- 1 tsp paprika
- 3 tbsp egg white
- Salt and pepper to taste

INSTRUCTIONS

1. Preheat air fryer to 200°C.
2. In a medium bowl, season shrimp with seasonings.
3. Place flour, breadcrumbs and egg in 3 separate dishes.

4. Dip shrimp in flour, egg lastly breadcrumb bread morsels.
5. Spray shrimp with cooking oil and place in air fryer container.
6. Cool for 4 minutes, flip and cook for an additional 4 minutes or until firm.

223. Air Fryer Pop Tarts

Total time: 25 minutes
Servings: 6

INGREDIENTS

- 2 pie crusts, refrigerated
- 1 tsp cornstarch
- 1/2 cup plain Greek yogurt
- 1/2 cup strawberry preserves
- 1 oz. Cream cheese
- Oil spray and some sugar sprinkles

INSTRUCTIONS

1. Place pie hulls on a level surface and utilizing a pizza shaper, cut outside layers into 6 rectangular shapes.
2. Add strawberry jam and cornstarch in a bowl and mix well.
3. Add 1 tbsp protect blend to the upper piece of the hull.
4. Fold outside layer to close the pop tarts and make engraves on every tart utilizing a fork.
5. Place pop tarts in air fryer container and splash with cooking oil.
6. Air fry at 190°C for 9 to 10 minutes or until sufficiently fresh just as you would prefer.
7. Combine Greek yogurt and cream cheese in a bowl to make an icing.
8. Top each pop tart with the icing and sprinkle sugar sprinkles over each.

224. Air Fryer Apple Dessert Empanadas

Total time: 32 minutes
Servings: 12

INGREDIENTS

- 12 empanada wrappers
- 2 tbsp raw honey
- 2 apples, diced
- 1 tsp cinnamon and vanilla extract
- 2 tsp cornstarch
- Cooking spray

INSTRUCTIONS

1. Place a skillet over medium warm. Include diced apples, cinnamon, honey, and vanilla.
2. Mix and cook for 3 minutes.
3. Add cornstarch in a bowl and blend in with water.
4. Add the blend to that skillet and cook for 30 seconds.
5. Place empanada wrappers on a level surface. Add the blend to every wrapper.
6. Roll empanada into equal parts, at that point roll every one of the side internal.
7. Keep on turning the moving sides until shut.
8. Add empanadas to the air fryer bin and fry at 200°C for 8 minutes.
9. Flip and cook for an additional 10 minutes.
10. Allow empanadas to cool before serving.

225.   Air Fryer Parmesan Truffle Fries

Total time: 40minutes
Servings: 4

INGREDIENTS

- 4 large russet potatoes
- 1/4 cup parmesan cheese
- 4 tsp oil
- 4 tsp fresh parsley
- 1 tsp paprika
- Salt and pepper

INSTRUCTIONS

1. Soak potatoes in a large bowl of cold water for around 30 minutes.
2. Drain and pat potatoes dry with paper towels.
3. Coat every potato with 1 tbsp of oil and seasonings. Separation in 2 equivalent segments.
4. Add first bit into the air fryer basket and cook at 190°C for 15 to 20 minutes.
5. Stop and shake at 10 minutes.
6. Add oil and parmesan cheese.
7. Sprinkle parsley over fries and serve!

226.   Air Fryer Grilled Cheese

Total time: 12 minutes
Servings: 1

INGREDIENTS

- 2 slices bread
- 1 tsp butter
- 2 slices cheddar cheese
- 1 tbsp turkey, optional
- Cooking spray

INSTRUCTIONS

1. Preheat air fryer to 175°C.
2. Spread butter on the 2 sides of bread. Add cheese and turkey between the two slices
3. Place sandwich in air fryer basket and cook for 5 minutes, turning halfway through.

227.   Air Fryer Cinnamon Rolls

Total time: 30minutes
Servings: 8

INGREDIENTS

- 1-pound frozen bread dough
- 1.5 tbsp cinnamon
- 1/2 cup butter
- 3/4 cup brown sugar
- 1/4 cups powdered sugar
- 4 oz. cream cheese
- Vanilla extract

INSTRUCTIONS

1. Roll mixture into a 13 by 11' square. Brush with melted butter.
2. Combine brown sugar and cinnamon in a bowl.
3. Sprinkle cinnamon blend liberally over buttered batter and roll firmly.
4. Press the revealed edge and seal firmly.
5. Let rolls sit at room temperature for around 2 hours.
6. For the coating, add cream cheese and butter to a bowl and microwave for around 30 seconds.
7. Mix in powdered sugar and vanilla concentrate. Whisk until smooth.
8. Preheat air fryer to 175°C. Place rolls in air fryer crate without covering.
9. Air fry for 5 minutes, turn and air fry for another 4 to 5 minutes.

228. Air Fryer S'mores

INGREDIENTS

- 4 graham crackers cut in half
- 4 tsp chocolate cream
- 1-pound strawberries
- 4 marshmallows
- Air fryers

INSTRUCTIONS

1. Preheat air fryer to 180°C.
2. Place 4 crackers in air fryer basket without overlapping and put 1 marshmallow on each biscuit
3. Cook for 5 minutes until caramelized and golden.
4. Add berries and chocolate cream and cover each with remaining crackers.

229. Glazed Salmon

Total time: 17 minutes
Servings: 4

INGREDIENTS

- 1-pound salmon fillet, deboned
- 1/4 cup Brown sugar
- 2 tbsp Dijon mustard
- Pepper
- Salt
- Parsley, optional

INSTRUCTIONS

1. Cut salmon into 4 portions.
2. Combine salt and pepper in a bowl and coat each side of salmon with salt-pepper mixture.
3. In another bowl, combine brown sugar and Dijon mustard.
4. Brush into salmon skin.
5. Place salmon in air fryer basket and air fry at 175°C for 15 minutes, skin side down.
6. Sprinkle with parsley and serve.

230. Air Fryer Garlic Parmesan Asparagus

Total time: 15 minutes
Servings: 4

INGREDIENTS

- 1-pound asparagus, washed and cut
- 1/2 tsp garlic powder
- 1/4 cup parmesan cheese
- 1/2 lemon
- 2 tsp olive oil
- Salt and pepper

INSTRUCTIONS

1. Toss asparagus in olive oil and garlic powder.
2. Add a pinch of salt and pepper. Squeeze lemon on asparagus and mix together to coat evenly.
3. Place in air fryer basket at 195°C for 10 minutes.
4. Sprinkle with cheese and enjoy!

231. Air Fryer Potatoes

Total time: 1 hour
Servings:

INGREDIENTS

- 1.5 pounds potatoes, washed and diced
- 1/2 tsp paprika
- 1/4 onion, chopped
- 1 green bell pepper, chopped
- 1 tbsp olive oil
- Salt and pepper

INSTRUCTIONS

1. Soak diced potatoes in water for 30 minutes. Pat dry with paper towels.
2. Place all ingredients including potatoes in a large bowl and mix together.
3. Toss into the air fryer basket and cook at 200°C for 10 minutes.
4. Shake basket and cook for another 10 minutes. Shake basket again and cook for 5 minutes more.
5. Serve and enjoy!

232. Air Fryer Pork Loin

Total time: 25 minutes
Servings: 6

INGREDIENTS

- 1.5 lb. pork tenderloins
- 2 small heads roasted garlic
- Salt
- Pepper
- Cooking spray

INSTRUCTIONS

1. Lightly coat all sides of pork tenderloins with cooking spray.
2. Coat with salt and pepper, then rub with roasted garlic.
3. Spray air fryer basket and place pork in. Cook at 200°C for 10 minutes.
4. Flip and add remaining garlic, and cook for another 10 minutes.
5. Let it rest for 5 minutes before serving with any veggies of your choice.

233. Air Fryer Coconut Shrimp

Total time: 15 minutes
Servings: 4

INGREDIENTS

- 1-pound large shrimp
- 1/2 cup all-purpose flour
- 1/2 tsp of baking powder
- 2 cups sweetened coconut, shredded
- 1/2 breadcrumbs
- Salt and 1 cup water

INSTRUCTIONS

1. In a medium bowl, combine flour, salt, water and baking powder and whisk together. Set aside.
2. In another medium bowl, blend breadcrumbs and coconut.
3. Dredge each shrimp in fluid flour blend and coat liberally in breadcrumb blend.
4. Preheat air fryer to 200°C and air fry for 5 minutes, without covering.

234. Air Fryer Roasted Chicken

Servings: 6

INGREDIENTS

- 1 whole chicken
- 2 tbsp Italian seasoning
- 3 tbsp avocado oil
- 2 tbsp chopped parsley
- 1 tsp garlic powder
- Salt and pepper

INSTRUCTIONS

1. In a large bowl, combine oil and Italian flavoring with garlic powder and cleaved parsley.
2. With your fingers, spread blend all over the chicken and sprinkle with salt and pepper.
3. Place in air fryer crate and cook for 30 minutes.

235. Air Fryer Sausage & Potatoes

Servings: 4

INGREDIENTS

- 1.5 lbs. small potatoes, golden
- 1 large onion, slices into large pieces
- 15 oz. sausage, sliced
- 2 tbsp olive oil
- 2 tbsp whole grain mustard mixed with honey
- Salt and pepper

INSTRUCTIONS

1. Toss onions and potatoes in oil, pepper, salt, and flavoring.
2. Place in air fryer crate and splash with cooking oil.
3. Air fry at 200°C for 15 to 16 minutes until delicate.
4. Shake crate part way through cooking.
5. Add sausage and cook for an additional 5 minutes.

236. Air Fryer Chicken Fried Rice

Total time: 40 minutes
Servings: 4

INGREDIENTS

- 3 cups white rice, cooked
- 1 cup diced chicken, also cooked
- 1 cup diced carrots, onions and peas
- 1 tbsp olive oil, or vegetable oil
- 6 tbsp soy sauce

INSTRUCTIONS

1. Place rice into a large bowl.
2. Add oil and soy sauce and mix together.
3. Add peas, carrots and diced onions. Add cooked chicken and mix thoroughly.

4. Pour mixture into a non-stick cooking pan and place the pan into the air fryer.
5. Cook at 160°C for 20 minutes, shaking halfway through.
6. Serve and enjoy!

237. Air Fryer Shrimp Fried Rice

Total time: 40 minutes
Servings: 4

INGREDIENTS

- 3 cups cooked white rice, frozen
- 1 cup shrimps, cleaned and cooked
- 1 cup diced carrots, onions and peas
- 6 tbsp soy sauce
- 1 tbsp vegetable oil

INSTRUCTIONS

1. Combine cooked white rice with vegetable oil and soy sauce in a large bowl and blend completely.
2. Add peas, diced carrots, onion, and shrimps and combine.
3. Spray skillet with non-stick cooking oil and empty rice-shrimp blend into the dish.
4. Place skillet into the air fryer and cook at 160°C for 20 minutes.

238. Air Fryer Steak Fries

Total time: 25 minutes
Servings: 6

INGREDIENTS

- 2 large russet potatoes
- 2 tbsp garlic, grated
- 1 tbsp olive oil
- 1/4 cup parmesan cheese, shredded
- Seasonings
- 1/4 tsp pepper, optional

INSTRUCTIONS

1. Slice potatoes into wedges and place in a bowl.
2. Drizzle with oil and mix with seasonings.
3. Transfer potatoes to air fryer bin and air fry at 200°C for 20 minutes.
4. Mix part of the way through.
5. Serve with ketchup or any dipping sauce.

239. Air Fryer Breakfast Burritos

Total time: 20 minutes
Servings: 6

INGREDIENTS

- 6 flour tortillas
- 6 eggs, scrambled
- 0.5 lb. sausage, browned
- 1/2 cup shredded cheese
- 1/2 red bell pepper, minced

INSTRUCTIONS

1. In a large bowl, combine sausage, eggs, bell pepper and cheese, and stir to mix properly.
2. Place about 3 tbsp of the mixture into the center of each tortilla dough.
3. Fold the sides in and roll.
4. Place burritos into air fryer basket and spray generously with cooking spray.
5. Air fry at 165°C for 5 minutes and serve.

240. Bacon-Wrapped Filet Mignon

Total time: 20 minutes
Servings: 1

INGREDIENTS

- 2 slices bacon
- 2 beef filets, cut into large pieces
- 1 tsp kosher salt
- Favorite seasoning
- Cooking spray

INSTRUCTIONS

1. Wrap bacon around the filet and at ease with a toothpick.
2. Combine salt and flavoring on a degree plate.
3. Rub filet-bacon, top and base, with flavoring.
4. Place in an air fryer bin and splash with oil.
5. Air fry at 180° C for 20 minutes, flipping part way through.
6. Serve with vegetables.

241. Air Fryer Garlic Bread

Total time: 15 minutes
Servings: 10 pieces

INGREDIENTS

- 1 loaf fresh bread

- 1 clove garlic, chopped
- 2 tbsp olive oil
- 3 tbsp butter
- 1/2 tsp parsley
- Salt

INSTRUCTIONS

1. Preheat air fryer to 200°C.
2. Slice bread portion into equal parts, the long way.
3. Combine all ingredients in a bowl and spread onto the bread.
4. Air fry in tinfoil for 10 minutes.

242. Air Fryer Stuffed Potatoes

Total time: 20 minutes
Servings: 4

INGREDIENTS

- 2 baked potatoes
- 1/4 cup whole milk
- 1/2 cup mozzarella cheese, shredded
- 1/2 tbsp butter
- 1/4 tsp dried parsley
- Salt and pepper

INSTRUCTIONS

1. Cut baked potatoes lengthwise, in half.
2. Scoop out potato from each half leaving the skin and a little bit of potato to hold stuffing.
3. Put scooped potato in a medium bowl and add butter, milk and seasoning. Mash together.
4. Add cheese and mix together.
5. Add mashed potatoes back into the almost empty skin and bake in an air fryer for 10 minutes. Stop baking when cheese is melted or lightly brown.
6. Sprinkle with parsley and enjoy.

243. Air Fryer Salmon

Total time: 15 minutes
Servings: 4

INGREDIENTS

- 2 pounds fresh salmon
- 1/2 tsp pepper
- 1 tsp chili powder
- 4 lime

- Parsley and salt

INSTRUCTIONS

1. Season salmon with chili powder, pepper and salt.
2. After flavoring the salmon, cut out 2 of the limes and squeeze over the salmon.
3. Place salmon in air fryer basket and set air fryer to 175°C. Let it cool for 8 minutes.
4. Salmon is ready once it reaches 145°F in the thickest part with a meat thermometer.
5. Slice open the rest of the line and squeeze the lime juice over salmon.
6. Garnish with parsley and enjoy!

244. Air Fryer Drumstick

Total time: 25 minutes
Servings: 4

INGREDIENTS

- 4 skinless chicken thighs, deboned
- 1 tbsp brown sugar
- 1/2 tsp paprika
- 1/2 tsp oregano
- 1/4 tsp pepper
- Salt to taste

INSTRUCTIONS

1. Rinse chicken thighs and pat dry with paper towels.
2. Mix collectively the solving and sprinkle it on the 2 sides of fowl thighs.
3. Place in the air fryer and cook at 175°C for 10 minutes.
4. Flip and cook for an additional 10 minutes.

245. Air Fryer Easy Burger

Total time: 20 minutes
Servings: 2

INGREDIENTS

- 0.5-pound ground beef
- 2 brioche buns
- 2 slices yellow cheese
- 1 tsp salt
- 1 tsp pepper

INSTRUCTIONS

1. Using your hand, form ground beef into patties.
2. Add salt and pepper to patties to season it.
3. Place patties into air fryer basket and air fry at 175°C for 8 minutes.
4. Flip and cook for another 8 minutes.
5. Before they're done, add cheese and cook until cheese melts.
6. Place in the center of your buns as in a sandwich.
7. Enjoy!

246.   Air Fryer Hot Dog

Total time: 18 minutes
Servings: 3

INGREDIENTS

- 3 hot dogs
- 1 tbsp mustard
- Chili
- Ketchup
- 3 buns

INSTRUCTIONS

1. Place hot dogs in air fryer crate and air fry at 150°C for 4 to 5 minutes.
2. Once done, place into buns.
3. Top with ketchup, chili, mustard or any garnish of your choice.

247.   Air Fryer Mini Chicken Pizza

Total time: 10 minutes
Servings: 2

INGREDIENTS

- 2 muffins (English muffin)
- 1/2 cup shredded chicken breast
- 1/2 cup tomato sauce
- Mozzarella cheese, shredded
- 1/4 cup sliced onions

INSTRUCTIONS

1. Preheat air fryer to 200°C.
2. Place each English muffins on a flat plate and top with tomato sauce, chicken breast, cheese and onions.

3. Transfer to air fryer basket and cook until cheese is melted.
4. Serve warm or cool and enjoy!

248.   Air Fryer Mini Bagel Pizza

Total time: 18 minutes
Servings: 2

INGREDIENTS

- 4 bagel buns
- 8 slices mozzarella cheese
- 1 tbsp oregano leaves
- Basil
- 8 cherry tomatoes
- Salt

INSTRUCTIONS

1. Slice cherry tomatoes in half.
2. Preheat air fryer to 220°C.
3. Place bagel buns on a level surface and top with mozzarella cheese, oregano, salt, basil, and tomatoes.
4. Place in air fryer basket and air fry for 8 to 10 minutes until cheese is melted.

249.   Air Fryer Steak & Mushrooms

Total time: 20 minutes
Servings: 4

INGREDIENTS

- 1 lb. sirloin steak or ribeye
- 2 tbsp Worcestershire sauce
- 2 tsp olive oil
- 8 oz. mushrooms, sliced
- 1 pack onion mix soup

INSTRUCTIONS

1. Cut steak into bite size portions and place in a large bowl.
2. Mix remaining ingredients and add to the steak.
3. Place steak with mushroom mixture into air fryer basket.
4. Air fry at 200°C for 10 to 13 minutes.
5. Serve and enjoy.

250.   Air Fryer Chicken & Black Bean Taquito

Total time: 20 minutes

Servings: 12

INGREDIENTS

- 1 1/2 cup shredded cooked chicken
- 1 cup shredded cheddar cheese
- 12 corn tortillas
- 1/2 cup salsa
- 1 can black beans, rinsed
- Cooking spray

INSTRUCTIONS

1. In a medium bowl, combine chicken, black beans and salsa and divide into 12 different parts for each tortilla.
2. Place each chicken mixture in the middle of corn tortillas and top with cheese.
3. Roll up tortillas and lightly press down the seams.
4. Place each tortilla into air fryer basket and spray with cooking spray.
5. Air fry at 200°C for 7 minutes. Repeat for all tortillas.
6. Serve and enjoy!

251.   Air Fryer Taco Ranch Bites

Total time: 20 minutes
Servings: 30 mini bites

INGREDIENTS

- 0.5 lb. ground beef
- 1/2 can diced tomatoes and green chili
- 1/2 bottle ranch seasoning
- 30 frozen tart shells
- 1 cup shredded Cheddar
- Taco seasoning

INSTRUCTIONS

1. In a saucer, cook beef until brown.
2. Add taco seasoning and diced tomatoes and mix. Cook for 5 to 6 minutes. Remove from heat.
3. Combine cheese, ranch dressing and taco beef.
4. Add mixture into frozen tart shells.
5. Preheat air fryer to 175°C and air fry for 8 minutes or until cheese has fully melted.
6. Serve and enjoy.

252.   Air Fryer Pita Bread Pizza

Total time: 12 minutes
Servings: 4

INGREDIENTS

- 4 pita breads
- 12 tbsp grated cheese
- 6 tbsp tomato sauce
- Olives
- Extra topping, optional

INSTRUCTIONS

1. Preheat air fryer to 180°C.
2. Spread tomato sauce on pita bread and sprinkle with cheese.
3. You can add your extra topping if using.
4. Line the bottom of air fryer basket with parchment paper.
5. Place bread pizza on top of parchment paper and air fry for 6 to 8 minutes.

253.   Air Fryer Popcorn

Total time: 20 minutes
Servings: 5

INGREDIENTS

- 3 tbsp dried corn kernels
- Salt
- 1 tsp dried chives
- Cooking spray
- 2 tbsp nutritional yeast
- Sugar, optional

INSTRUCTIONS

1. Preheat air fryer to 200°C.
2. Add kernels to air fryer basket and spray with cooking spray or avocado oil.
3. Place basket into air fryer and air fry for 15 minutes.
4. Check every 4 minutes to prevent burning.
5. Remove basket and pour contents into a large bowl.
6. Spray lightly with cooking spray and sprinkle with yeast, chives and sugar, if using.
7. Serve and enjoy!

254.   Air Fryer Garnished Pancake

Total time: 15 minutes

Servings: 5

INGREDIENTS

- 1 cup whole wheat flour
- 3 large eggs, beaten
- 1 cup almond milk
- Confectioners' sugar
- Fresh berries
- Salt

INSTRUCTIONS

1. Preheat air fryer to 200°C and set iron tray inside.
2. Combine flour, eggs, almond milk and a pinch of salt to form batter and mix until well blended.
3. Spray iron tray with cooking spray and pour in the batter.
4. Air fry for 6 to 8 minutes.
5. Garnish with confectioners' sugar and berries and enjoy!

255.   Air Fryer Cinnamon Toast

Total time: 15 minutes
Servings: 3

INGREDIENTS

- 6 slices whole wheat bread
- 1/2 stick butter
- 1/4 cup white sugar
- 3/4 tsp ground cinnamon
- 3/4 tsp vanilla extract
- Salt

INSTRUCTIONS

1. In a bowl, place butter and add in sugar, cinnamon, salt and vanilla extract. Mix well.
2. Spread mixture onto the surface of the bread.
3. Place bread slices in air fryer basket and air fry at 200°C for 5 minutes.
4. Remove and cut diagonally.
5. Serve warm.

256.   Air Fryer Mini Cheese Scones

Total time: 30 minutes
Servings: 5

INGREDIENTS

- 90g flour
- Butter
- 1/2 egg, beaten
- 1 cup Cheddar
- 1/2 tbsp whole milk
- Mustard and chives
- Salt and pepper

INSTRUCTIONS

1. In a large bowl, combine flour and butter until well blended.
2. Add in spices and half of the cheese.
3. Add milk and egg, mixing well.
4. Roll out batter and partition into 5 equivalent segments.
5. Place remaining cheese at the center point of every batter and make it into balls.
6. Preheat air fryer 180°C.
7. Place mini-scones in the air fryer basket and cook for 20 minutes.

257.   Air Fryer Garlic Croutons

Servings: 4

INGREDIENTS

- 4 slices whole wheat bread
- 2 tbsp olive oil
- 1 tsp garlic powder
- 1 tsp salt
- Cooking spray, optional

INSTRUCTIONS

1. Cut bread into cubes and toss with olive oil.
2. Sprinkle with some garlic powder and salt.
3. Place bread cubes in air fryer basket and air fry at 200°C for 5 to 8 minutes.
4. Shake basket halfway through frying.
5. Serve and enjoy.

258.   Air Fryer Flourless Crispy Calamari Rings

Total time: 15 minutes
Servings: 2

INGREDIENTS

- 1 cup plain oats
- 1 large egg, beaten

- 2/3 lb. calamari
- 1 small lemon
- 1 tbsp paprika
- Salt and pepper to taste

INSTRUCTIONS

1. Slice calamari into rings.
2. Blend oats until particles are fine. Place in a bowl and mix in spices.
3. Place beaten eggs in another bowl.
4. Coat calamari rings in salt and pepper and lemon juice.
5. Then place them into oats, place in eggs lastly in oats again to cover liberally.
6. Place in air fryer bin and cook at 180°C for 8 minutes.
7. Serve and enjoy.

259.   Air Fryer Pig-In-The-Blanket

Total time: 20 minutes
Servings: 6

INGREDIENTS

- 6 bacon slices
- 2 large sausages
- Salt
- Pepper
- Cooking spray

INSTRUCTIONS

1. Chop sausages into 3 equal portions.
2. Wrap each sausage in the bacon.
3. Spray air fryer basket with cooking spray.
4. Place wrapped sausage in air fryer basket and air fry at 180°C for 15 minutes.
5. Sprinkle with salt and pepper and serve.

260.   Air Fryer Garlic Roasted Mushrooms

Total time: 40 minutes
Servings: 2

INGREDIENTS

- 1-pound mushrooms, washed
- 1 tsp white vermouth
- 1/4 tbsp garlic powder
- 1/2 tbsp goose fat
- 1 tbsp herbs de Provence

INSTRUCTIONS

1. Spin dry mushroom in salad spinner. Cut them into quarters and set aside.
2. Put goose fat, garlic powder, and herbs in the pan of your air fryer.
3. Air fry for 2 minutes, add mushrooms and cook for another 25 minutes.
4. After 25 minutes, add white vermouth and cook for another 5 minutes.
5. Serve and enjoy.

261.   Air Fryer Turkey Burger

Total time: 50 minutes
Servings: 4

INGREDIENTS

- 1 lb. ground turkey
- 1/2 onion grated
- 1 tbsp ranch seasoning
- 2 tsp Worcestershire sauce
- 1/2 cup breadcrumbs
- Salt and pepper to taste

INSTRUCTIONS

1. In a medium bowl, combine turkey, ranch seasoning, onions, Worcestershire sauce, salt and pepper, and breadcrumbs.
2. Mix properly with your hands.
3. Divide mixture into 4 hamburger patties of equal size.
4. Place burgers in the refrigerator and leave them to firm up for about 30 minutes.
5. Preheat Air Fryer to 180°C.
6. Place burger patties in Air fryer without overlapping.
7. Cook for 15 minutes, flipping halfway through.
8. Serve and enjoy.

262.   Air Fryer Fish

Total time: 30 minutes
Servings: 4

INGREDIENTS

- 5 Fish fillets cut in half and rinsed
- 1 cup fine cornmeal
- 2 tsp old bay
- 1 tsp paprika
- 1/2 tsp garlic powder

- Salt and pepper to taste

INSTRUCTIONS

1. Pat fish fillets dry with paper towels.
2. Place filets in Ziploc baggie and shake until totally ensured.
3. Oil or sprinkle the base of the air fryer box with a cooking, washing, at that factor place the filets inside the receptacle.
4. Flip and get ready supper the elective aspect for 7 minutes.
5. Remove and serve.

263. Air Fryer Chili Lime Chickpeas

Total time: 23 minutes
Servings: 3

INGREDIENTS

- 1 can Garbanzo beans, drained
- 1 tsp chili powder
- 1/4 tsp garlic powder
- 1/4 tsp lime juice
- 1/4 tsp cumin
- 1/4 tsp salt

INSTRUCTIONS

1. Preheat air fryer to 200°C and place chickpeas in air Fryer basket.
2. Spray with cooking oil and air fry for 18 minutes, shaking every 5 minutes.
3. When there's 2 minutes left, open air fryer and sprinkle half of the seasoning on the chickpeas.
4. Air fry for the remaining 2 minutes.
5. Remove and place in a bowl, then sprinkle remaining seasoning on the chickpeas and toss to combine.
6. Serve and enjoy.

264. Air Fryer Honey Mustard Pork Chops

Total time: 18 minutes
Servings: 4

INGREDIENTS

- 1 lb. boneless pork chops, center-cut
- 1 tsp yellow mustard
- 2 tsp raw honey
- 1 tsp steak seasoning blend

- Cooking spray, optional

INSTRUCTIONS

1. In a bowl, combine mustard, honey, and steak flavoring mix and blend well.
2. Using a brush, add mustard blend to the 2 sides of pork cleaves for covering.
3. Place pork in a single layer in the air fryer bin.
4. Set air fryer to 180°C and air fry for 12 minutes, flipping partially through.

265. Air Fryer Stuffed Chicken Breast

Total time: 30 minutes
Servings: 2

INGREDIENTS

- 6 oz. boneless skinless chicken breasts
- 1/2 cup wild rice, prepared
- 2 oz. Feta Cheese
- 2 tbsp Greek Salad Dressing
- Parsley, optional

INSTRUCTIONS

1. Cut the chicken breasts into half to get 2 portions.
2. Pound chicken breasts until thin.
3. In a small bowl, combine prepared wild rice, Greek dressing and Feta cheese.
4. Place 1/2 of the rice mixture onto the center of each chicken breast and roll over the mixture.
5. Place chicken breasts side down into air fryer baking pan.
6. Brush chicken breasts with remaining Greek dressing.
7. Cook at 190°C for 13 to 15 minutes.
8. Serve and enjoy!

266. Air Fryer Tuna Cake

Total time: 20 minutes
Servings: 2

INGREDIENTS

- 2 cans tuna, drained
- 1 tbsp all-purpose flour
- 1 tsp mayonnaise
- 1/4 tsp garlic powder
- 1/4 tsp black pepper

- Salt to taste

INSTRUCTIONS

1. In a small bowl, combine fish, flour, mayonnaise, garlic powder, dark pepper and salt and mix well.
2. Divide into 4 equal pieces and form small patties.
3. Air fry at 190°C for 10 minutes, flipping partially through.
4. Serve and enjoy!

267. Air Fryer Roasted Turkey Breast

Total time: 1hour 10minutes
Servings: 4

INGREDIENTS

- 3 pounds boneless turkey breast
- 2 tsp poultry seasoning
- 1/2 tsp garlic powder
- 1/4 tsp black pepper
- 1/4 cup mayonnaise
- Salt to taste

INSTRUCTIONS

1. Preheat air fryer to 180°C.
2. Rub and season turkey breast with mayonnaise, poultry flavoring, garlic powder, dark pepper, and salt.
3. Place in Air fryer container and air fry for 60 minutes, checking and turning at regular intervals.
4. Serve and enjoy it.

268. Turkey Thighs

Total time: 50minutes
Servings: 2

INGREDIENTS

- 2 large turkey thighs
- 1 tsp brown sugar
- 1/2 tsp garlic powder
- 1 tbsp paprika
- Cooking spray
- Salt to taste

INSTRUCTIONS

1. In a bowl, combine brown sugar, garlic powder, paprika and salt until well mixed.
2. Rinse turkey thighs in water and pat dry with a paper towel.
3. On a flat surface, rub seasoning all over turkey thighs and also under the skin.
4. Place turkey in air fryer basket and spray lightly with cooking spray.
5. Air fry at 200°C for 20 minutes. Flip and cook for another 20 minutes.
6. Remove and serve.

269. Air Fryer Home Fries

Total time: 30minutes
Servings: 2

INGREDIENTS

- 3 large potatoes
- 1 tbsp olive oil
- Salt
- Pepper
- Ketchup

INSTRUCTIONS

1. Cut potatoes with potatoes shaper, into strips.
2. Place potatoes in water and add salt Soak for around 45 minutes.
3. Drain and pat dry with a paper towel.
4. Sprinkle with some pepper, if using and place in air fryer basket. Grease with cooking oil.
5. Cook fries for 25 minutes, flipping halfway through.

270. Air Fryer Roasted Carrots

Total time: 15 minutes
Servings: 4

INGREDIENTS

- 3 cups carrots, sliced into large chunks
- 1 tbsp raw honey
- 1 tbsp olive oil
- Salt
- Pepper

INSTRUCTIONS

1. In a bowl, combine carrots, honey and olive oil.

2. Season with salt and pepper and ensure they are well coated.
3. Transfer to air fryer and cook at 200° for 12 minutes.
4. Serve hot and enjoy.

271. Air Fryer Shoestring Carrots

Total time: 20 minutes
Servings: 2

INGREDIENTS

- 10 oz. julienned carrots
- 1 tbsp olive oil
- 1 tsp orange zest
- Apple cider vinegar
- Salt and pepper

INSTRUCTIONS

1. In a bowl, combine carrots with olive oil and coat lightly.
2. Season to taste with salt and pepper.
3. Place seasoned carrots in air fryer basket and cook at 200°C for 14 to 16 minutes.
4. Shake basket every 5 minutes.
5. Stop cooking when carrots are nicely brown.
6. Remove from air fryer and place in a serving bowl.
7. Add orange zest, spray with a little apple cider vinegar and re-season with salt and pepper if needed.
8. Serve hot.

272. Air Fryer Parsnip Fries

Total time: 15 minutes
Servings: 2

INGREDIENTS

- 1 lb. parsnips
- 1 tbsp olive oil
- 1 tsp salt
- 1 tsp pepper
- 2 tsp corn flour

INSTRUCTIONS

1. Cut parsnips as uniformly as possible. Place in a bowl.
2. Add in olive oil, salt and pepper.

3. Then add corn flour and shake gently to ensure an even coating.
4. Place parsnips in air fryer basket and cook for 180°C for 10 minutes.
5. Increase temperature to 190°C for another 4 minutes, shaking basket halfway through.
6. Remove when fries become brown and adjust seasoning if needed.
7. Serve and enjoy!

273. Air Fryer Zucchini, Squash & Carrots

Total time: 45minutes
Servings: 3-4

INGREDIENTS

- 1/2 lb. carrots, peeled and cut into cubes
- 1 lb. zucchini, peeled and cut into half moons
- 1 lb. yellow squash, trimmed and cut into half moons
- 5 tbsp olive oil
- 1 tbsp tarragon leaves, chopped
- Salt and white pepper

INSTRUCTIONS

1. In a bowl, combine carrots and 2 spoonfuls of olive oil and toss together.
2. Place carrots in the air fryer basket and cook at 200°C for 5 minutes.
3. Meanwhile place zucchini and squash in another bowl and grease with staying olive oil.
4. Season with salt and pepper and toss.
5. Add zucchini and squash to the carrots in the basket and cook for an additional 30 minutes, shaking twice all through cooking.
6. Remove from air fryer and toss with tarragon leaves.
7. Serve and enjoy it.

274. Air Fryer French Green Beans

Total time: 25 minutes
Servings: 5

INGREDIENTS

- 1.5 lb. French green beans
- 2 tbsp olive oil
- 1/2 lb. shallots, scraped, stem discarded and cut into quarters
- 1/2 tsp white pepper
- 1/4 cup slivered almonds, toasted

- Salt to taste

INSTRUCTIONS

1. Boil green beans and 1 tbsp salt for 3 minutes. Drain water.
2. Place in a large bowl with shallots, 1 tsp of salt, white pepper, and olive oil.
3. Coat well.
4. Place in air fryer crate and cook at 200°C for 25 minutes, tossing part of the way through cooking.

275. Air Fryer Lemony Green Beans

Total time: 10 minutes
Servings: 4

INGREDIENTS

- 1 lb. green beans, destemmed
- 1 lemon
- 1/4 tsp olive oil
- Salt
- Black pepper

INSTRUCTIONS

1. Place green beans in air fryer basket.
2. Add few drops of lemon juice.
3. Add salt and pepper to taste.
4. Drizzle olive oil over the top.
5. Cook for 200°C for 10 to 14 minutes depending on your taste.
6. Serve and enjoy.

276. Air Fryer Breaded Raviolis

Total time: 45 minutes
Servings: 6

INGREDIENTS

- 6 pre-made cheese ravioli
- 2 small eggs, beaten
- 1 cup flour
- 1 cup breadcrumbs
- Marinara sauce

INSTRUCTIONS

1. Place beat eggs, flour and bread morsels in 3 separate dishes.

2. Dip every ravioli in egg bowl, in flour, over into egg lastly in bread morsels to cover appropriately.
3. Place in air fryer container and cook at 185°C for 18 to 20 minutes.

277. Air Fryer Zucchini Zircles

Total time: 25 minutes
Servings: 3

INGREDIENTS

- 3 large zucchinis, cut into 1/4 inch thick
- 1/2 cup all-purpose flour
- 1/2 cup powdered sugar
- 1 cup milk
- 1 cup Italian breadcrumbs

INSTRUCTIONS

1. Place zucchini on lined baking sheet.
2. Place flour, milk and prepared bread morsels in 3 separate dishes.
3. Coat zucchini in flour, place in milk and afterward in bread morsels.
4. Gently place zucchini hovers in lubed air fryer bin and grease with cooking oil.
5. Cook at 200°C for 8 minutes, flipping part of the way through.
6. Remove from air fryer and sprinkle powdered sugar over it.
7. Serve with any dipping sauce of your choice.

278. Air Fryer Tomato and Onion Quiche

Total time: 35 minutes
Servings: 1

INGREDIENTS

- 1/4 cup milk
- 2 eggs
- 1/2 cup cheese, shredded
- 1/4 cup tomatoes, diced
- 1/4 diced onions
- Salt to taste

INSTRUCTIONS

1. Place all ingredients in a bowl and whisk together.
2. Place in air fryer basket and cook at 170°C for 30 minutes.

3. Remove and serve warm.

279. Air Fryer Cheese Stick Egg Rolls

Total time: 45 minutes

Servings: 24

INGREDIENTS

- 2 packs sliced steak, frozen
- 1 pack egg roll wrappers
- 1 white onion, diced
- 1 green bell pepper, diced
- 1/2 lb. cheese

INSTRUCTIONS

1. Heat a pot and grease with olive oil. Include vegetables until cooked yet at the same time fresh.
2. Remove from the pot onto a paper towel-lined plate.
3. Still in past pot, cook a steak so the flavor structure vegetable can blend in with the steak.
4. Add a place of salt to the meat or to taste and separate the meat into pieces with a wooden spatula.
5. Allow meat to cook for 10 to 15 minutes or until not pink any longer. Remove and allow to cool.
6. In a large bowl, combine cooked meat, cheese, and precooked vegetables. Mix well to combine.
7. Place egg move wrappers on a level surface and place 1/4 of your filling into the middle.
8. Turn edges over filling and overlap the creases.
9. Transfer egg folds into air fryer crate and cook at 175°C for 10 minutes and another 196°C for 3 minutes.
10. Remove and serve.

280. Thai Peanut Chicken Egg Rolls

Total time: 20 minutes

Servings: 4

INGREDIENTS

- 4 egg roll wrappers
- 2 cups shredded rotisserie chicken
- 1/4 cup Thai peanut sauce
- 3 green onions, chopped

- 1/4 red bell pepper, chopped
- non-stick cooking spray

INSTRUCTIONS

1. Preheat Air fryer to 195°C.
2. In a bowl, blend chicken in with Thai shelled nut sauce.
3. Place egg move wrappers on a level and dry surface.
4. Orchestrate ¼ carrot, bell pepper and onions at the base of an egg move wrapper.
5. At that point spoon 1/2 cup of the chicken blend on the vegetables.
6. To the outside edges of the wrapper, saturate with your hand dunked in water.
7. Crease the edges towards the inside and roll firmly.
8. Repeat with residual egg move wrappers.
9. Spray egg moves on the 2 sides with a non-stick cooking oil.
10. Place them in the Air fryer and air fryer at 190°C for 6-8 minutes until fresh and brilliant dark-colored.
11. Serve and enjoy it.

281. Air Fryer Avocado Corn Chicken Nachos

Total time: 22 minutes

Servings:

INGREDIENTS

- 3 cups tortilla chips
- 1 cup chicken, shredded
- 1 cup pepper jack cheese, shredded
- 1 cup Avocado Corn Salsa
- Cooking spray

INSTRUCTIONS

1. Preheat air fryer to 175°C.
2. Place tortilla chips on a sheet and top with shredded chicken and cheese. Spray with cooking spray.
3. Transfer to air fryer basket and air fry for 10 minutes.
4. Top the nachos with Avocado Corn Salsa.
5. Serve immediately and enjoy.

282. Air Fryer Buffalo Cauliflower Tots

Total time: 30 minutes

Servings: 4

INGREDIENTS

- 16 oz frozen cauliflower tots
- 3 tbsp buffalo wing sauce
- Cheese crumbles and celery sticks, optional
- Ranch dressing, optional

INSTRUCTIONS

1. Place frozen cauliflower tots in Air fryer basket and cook at 195°C for 20 minutes, tossing halfway through cooking.
2. Place cooked tots in a bowl and toss with buffalo sauce until they have been well coated.
3. Return tots to the Air fryer and air fry for another 5 minutes.
4. Serve hot with cheese crumbles, celery and/or ranch dressing.

283.   Air Fryer Low Carb Pickles

Total time: 37 minutes
Servings: 7

INGREDIENTS

- 1 large egg, whisked with 3/4 cup heavy cream
- 2 tbsp black pepper
- 35 dill pickle slices
- 4 cups pork rinds
- 1/2 cup almond flour
- 2 tbsp paprika, optional

INSTRUCTIONS

1. In a food processor, blend pork rinds.
2. Place half of the pork rind in a bowl and mix the remaining half with almond flour, paprika and black pepper.
3. Place egg-cream mixture in another bowl.
4. Dip each pickle first in pork rinds, then in egg mixture and finally in almond flour until well coated.
5. In batches, air fry pickles without overlapping at 190°C for 10 minutes or until golden brown.
6. Serve immediately with ranch dressing or any dipping sauce of your choice.

284.   Air Fryer Hot Prawn and Cocktail Sauce

Total time: 20 minutes
Servings: 4

INGREDIENTS

- 2 tsp chili flakes
- 10 fresh king prawns
- 3 tbsp mayonnaise
- 1 tbsp ketchup sauce
- 1 tsp wine vinegar
- Salt and ground black pepper

INSTRUCTIONS

1. Preheat the air fryer to 180°C.
2. Mix spices in a bowl and add prawns to coat.
3. Place coated prawns into the air fryer basket and air fry for 6 to 8 minutes, depending on prawn size.
4. Mix the ketchup and cocktail sauce in a bowl.

285.   Air Fryer Apricot and Blackberry Crumble

Total time: 30 minutes
Servings: 4

INGREDIENTS

- 100g all-purpose flour
- 250g fresh apricots
- 75g sugar
- 100g fresh blackberries
- 50g butter
- 1 tbsp lemon juice, optional

INSTRUCTIONS

1. Preheat air fryer to 200°C.
2. Remove pit from apricot and cut into cubes.
3. Place them in a bowl and mix with lemon juice, blackberries and 1/3 of the sugar.
4. Grease a 16cm diameter cake tin and spread fruit mix over the tin.
5. In another bowl, mix flour, a pinch of salt, remaining sugar, butter, and few drops of water until consistent.
6. Crumble with your fingers.
7. Scatter crumbly mixture evenly over the fruit mix.
8. Place tin in air fryer basket and air fry for 20 minutes or until golden brown.
9. Serve with ice cream.

286.   Air Fryer Roasted Lamb Rack

Total time: 40minutes
Servings: 4

INGREDIENTS

- 800g rack of lamb
- 75g almonds, chopped
- 1 tbsp breadcrumbs
- 1 clove chopped garlic mixed with olive oil
- 1 egg
- Salt and pepper

INSTRUCTIONS

1. Preheat air fryer to 100°C.
2. Brush garlic oil over the rack of lamb and season with salt and pepper.
3. Place almonds in a bowl and mix in breadcrumbs.
4. Whisk egg in another bowl.
5. Dip meat first into the egg blend, at that point in almond blend and coat liberally.
6. Place in the air fryer container. Air fry for 25 minutes.
7. Increase the temperature to 200°C and air fry for an additional 5 minutes.

287.   Air Fryer Double Cheeseburger
Total time: 28 minutes
Servings: 2

INGREDIENTS

- 2 Burger Buns
- 250g pork mince
- 1 onion-half diced; half sliced
- 50g cheddar cheese
- 1 tbsp soft cheese
- Salt and Pepper

INSTRUCTIONS

1. Preheat air fryer to 180°C.
2. Place pork mince, diced onion, salt & pepper and the soft cheese into a bowl.
3. Mix properly so that all ingredients are well combined and you have a large meatball.
4. Divide meatballs into 4 equal sized patties and place in preheated air fryer.
5. Cook for 10 minutes.
6. Remove, sprinkle with cheese and cook with reduced temperature for another 5 minutes.
7. When burgers are about 5 minutes from being ready, put sliced onion in a saucer and with some olive oil and allow to sauté.

8. When burger is ready, place salad garnish on the bun, followed by a burger, then press the other burger on top.
9. Sprinkle burger with some more cheese and fried onions.

288.   Air Fryer Lamb Burger
Total time: 22 minutes
Servings: 4

INGREDIENTS

- 600g minced lamb
- 2 tsp sautéed garlic
- 1 tbsp Harissa paste
- 1 tbsp spice
- Salt and Pepper

INSTRUCTIONS

1. Place minced lamb, garlic, paste, spices, salt and pepper in a bowl and mix well until lamb mince is seasoned.
2. Press mince into burger shape.
3. You can use a burger press.
4. Place lamb burgers in the air fryer basket and air fry at 180°C for 18 minutes.

289.   Air Fryer Jamaican Meatballs
Total time: 20 minutes
Servings: 4

INGREDIENTS

- 2 tbsp Jerk Dry Rub
- 100g mince chicken
- 100g breadcrumbs
- 4 tbsp raw honey
- 1 tbsp soy sauce

INSTRUCTIONS

1. In a bowl, place chicken and add breadcrumbs and 1 tbsp Jerk dry rub seasoning. Mix properly and press into meatball shapes, using a meatball press.
2. Place in the air fryer and cook at 180°C for 15 minutes.
3. In a mixing bowl, combine soy sauce, honey and remaining jerk seasoning and mix well.
4. When meatballs are done, dip or toss them in the sauce and serve.

290. Air Fryer Jacket Potatoes

Total time: 25 minutes
Servings: 2

INGREDIENTS

- 2 potatoes
- 50ml sour cream
- 1 tsp butter
- 25g cheese, grated
- Chives
- Salt & Pepper

INSTRUCTIONS

1. Stick a fork into potatoes and place them in air Fryer to cook for 15 minutes at 180°C.
2. Combine sour cream, cheese and chives in a bowl, until evenly mixed.
3. When the potatoes are done, pinch them open and spread with butter and filling mix.

291. Hasselback Potatoes

Total time: 30 minutes
Servings: 2

INGREDIENTS

- 2 Large Potatoes
- 1/2 tbsp Olive Oil
- 1/2 tbsp Parsley
- 1/2 tbsp rosemary
- 10g Cheddar
- Salt & Pepper

INSTRUCTIONS

1. Chop the potatoes.
2. Sprinkle with salt, pepper, and parsley and place in the air fryer for 20 minutes.
3. Mix olive oil and rosemary in a bowl.
4. Spread mix all over potatoes. Sprinkle with cheese.
5. Move to air fryer and cook for an extra 10 minutes.

292. Air Fryer Potato Gratin

Total time: 30 minutes
Servings: 2

INGREDIENTS

- 1 large potato
- 1 egg, beaten
- 50ml Coconut Cream
- 1/2 tbsp flour
- 25g cheddar

INSTRUCTIONS

1. Thinly slice potatoes (without peeling skin) and place in Air Fryer basket.
2. Cook at 180°C for 10 minutes or until crispy.
3. Meanwhile, combine eggs, coconut cream and flour until they have reached a thick consistency.
4. Remove potatoes from air fryer.
5. Line them in the bottom of 2 ramekins.
6. Cover ramekins with cream mixture, sprinkle with some cheese and cook for another 10 minutes at 200°C.
7. Serve and enjoy!

293. Coated Fish Sticks

Total time: 15 minutes
Servings: 3

INGREDIENTS

- 9 Fish Sticks
- 1 tsp Pepper
- 1 tsp Salt
- Olive oil spray
- 1/2 lime

INSTRUCTIONS

1. Remove frozen fish sticks
2. Pat dry with paper towels and spray with cooking spray.
3. Toss fish stick with salt and pepper and place in air fryer basket.
4. Air fry at 180°C for 8 minutes.
5. Remove from air fryer and drizzle with lime.
6. Serve and enjoy.

294. Air Fryer Fish Cake

Total time: 1 hour
Servings: 4

INGREDIENTS

- 3 cups cooked white fish

- 3 tbsp Milk
- 1 cup mashed potatoes
- 4 tsp butter
- 3 tbsp flour
- 1 Tsp Parsley, optional
- Salt & Pepper

INSTRUCTIONS

1. Combine potatoes, fish and seasoning in a large bowl and mix properly.
2. Add butter and milk and mix.
3. Add in little flour and form patties.
4. Refrigerate for about 3 hours to solidify patties.
5. Place in the Air Fryer and cook at 200°C for 15 minutes.
6. Serve and enjoy.

295.   Air Fryer Shortbread Cookies
Total time: 26 minutes
Servings: 2

INGREDIENTS

- 250g all-purpose flour
- 175g Butter
- 1 tbsp vanilla extract
- 70g caster sugar
- Black and white chocolate chips

INSTRUCTIONS

1. Preheat the air fryer to 180 C.
2. In a mixing bowl, combine flour, sugar and vanilla concentrate, then mix in the butter and blend until smooth.
3. Form cookies and place on a baking sheet. Air fry at 180° C for 10 minutes.
4. Halfway thru, fold the chocolate chips into the treats.
5. Cook for 10 more minutes.

296.   Air Fryer Chicken for Tacos
Total time: 30 minutes
Servings: 4

INGREDIENTS

- 500g chicken breasts
- 4 tbsp taco seasoning
- 1 tbsp olive oil

- 1 tbsp lime, juiced
- Salt & Pepper

INSTRUCTIONS

1. Place chicken, olive oil and taco seasoning in a Ziploc bag and shake well until well combined.
2. Place bag in a refrigerator for 2 hours to marinate.
3. After 2 hours, remove chicken from Ziploc bag and place in a baking dish.
4. Add taco seasoning on top and season with salt and pepper.
5. Transfer chicken breasts to the air fryer and cook at 180°C for 25 minutes.
6. Serve and enjoy.

297.   Air Fryer Pumpkin Seeds
Total time: 25 minutes
Servings: 6

INGREDIENTS

- 2 cups fresh pumpkin seeds, cleaned
- 1/2 tsp garlic powder
- 1 1/2 tbsp butter
- Salt
- Water

INSTRUCTIONS

1. Harvest seeds directly from pumpkin and wash with water.
2. Bring a pot of water to boil over medium heat, then place seeds in boiling water.
3. Boil for 5 minutes and drain.
4. Place boiled seeds in a bowl and add butter. Toss with garlic and salt.
5. Transfer seeds to air fryer and cook at 180°C for 15 minutes.
6. Serve and enjoy.

298.   Air Fryer Asparagus Pastry Twist
Total time: 25 minutes
Servings:

INGREDIENTS

- 24 Asparagus Spears
- 1 tbsp Extra Virgin Olive Oil
- Salt & Black Pepper
- 1 Pre-Rolled Puff Pastry Sheet

- 1 Egg
- ½ cup Parmesan Cheese, shredded/grated

INSTRUCTIONS

1. Rinse the asparagus under running water. Cut the ends off.
2. Place the cut asparagus skewers in a wide bowl.
3. Grease with olive oil and season with salt and pepper.
4. Unfold the puff pastry sheet. Cut it into about ½ inch (1.5 cm) strips.
5. Take a strip and fold it over asparagus stick, leaving some free space in the middle.
6. Leave the tip free.
7. Place onto a baking sheet lined with parchment paper.
8. Beat the egg in a bowl.
9. Brush the pastry of each asparagus twist with the egg wash and sprinkle with Parmesan cheese.
10. Bake in a preheated broiler at 400°F/200°C for 10 minutes.

299.   **Mango Chicken Puff**
Total time: 25 minutes
Servings: 10

INGREDIENTS

- 500g precooked Chicken Breasts, chopped
- 5 tbsp Mayonnaise
- 5 tbsp Mango Chutney
- 1 pre-Rolled Puff Pastry Sheet
- 1/3 cup Fresh Parsley, chopped
- 1 small egg, beaten

INSTRUCTIONS

1. Preheat air fryer to 180°C.
2. Cut puff pastry sheet into square shapes and place in the air fryer bin.
3. Brush them with egg wash.
4. Bake the puff pastry for 15 minutes.
5. Meanwhile mix chicken with mayonnaise, parsley and mango chutney.
6. Once puff pastry is prepared, let t cool.
7. Cut each piece down the middle.
8. Load with mango-chicken mix.

300.   **Air Fryer Bacon Pinwheel**
Total: 25 minutes
Servings: 12

INGREDIENTS

- 1 pre-rolled puff pastry sheet
- 4 tbsp Ketchup
- 7 oz bacon slices
- Thai sweet chili Sauce
- 1 cup cheddar, shredded

INSTRUCTIONS

1. Preheat air fryer to 200°C.
2. Unfold puff pastry sheet and spread ketchup over it.
3. Arrange the bacon slices to cover the entire pastry sheet.
4. Sprinkle with cheese and chili sauce.
5. Take the long edge of the pastry and move them. Cut into 0.5-inch pieces.
6. Transfer to air fryer bin and prepare for 20 minutes.

301.   **Air Fryer Cheeseball Bites**
Total time: 30 minutes
Servings: 30

INGREDIENTS

- 1 Celery Stick, finely chopped
- 1 Large Apple, finely chopped
- 1.4 oz Walnuts
- 1.7 oz Gouda Cheese
- 7 oz cream cheese
- For coating the balls:
- 3.5 oz Walnuts
- 3.5 oz Gouda Cheese

INSTRUCTIONS

1. Mix all ingredients: in a bowl and blend using a spoon/fork.
2. Coat half of them with finely hacked pecans and the other half with gouda.
3. Refrigerate for 30 minutes.

302.   **Hot Dog Mummies**
Total time: 27 minutes
Servings:

INGREDIENTS

- 12 Hot Dogs
- 1 pre-rolled Puff Pastry Sheet
- 24 Tiny Edible Sugar Eyes
- 1 tsp Mayo/Mustard/Ketchup

INSTRUCTIONS

1. Unroll the puff pastry. Cut it into strips.
2. Pat dry each sausage with a paper towel.
3. Wrap the puff pastry around the sausages, making a point to leave a hole for the eyes.
4. Bake them in a preheated stove at 360°F/180°C for 12-15 minutes.
5. Let them cool somewhat before putting the eyes on.
6. To do this, simply put a little mayo/ketchup/mustard on the posterior of the eye and adhere to the sausage.

303. Chicken Wings

Total time: 20 minutes
Servings: 4

INGREDIENTS

- 500g chicken wings
- 2 tbsp soy sauce
- 2 tbsp oyster sauce
- Black pepper
- Cooking spray
- Salt

INSTRUCTIONS

1. Preheat air fryer to 200°C.
2. Season wings with salt and black pepper.
3. Then add soy sauce and oyster sauce until well coated.
4. Place in preheated air fryer and spray with cooking spray.
5. Cook for 18 to 20 minutes, turning halfway through.
6. Serve warm and enjoy.

304. Air Fryer Mashed Potato Cake

INGREDIENTS

- 2 cups mashed potatoes
- 1/2 cup flour

- 2 eggs
- 1/4 cup sour cream
- Cooking spray

INSTRUCTIONS

1. Combine potatoes, flour and eggs in a bowl and mix well.
2. Shape into 12 patties.
3. Refrigerate patties for 30 minutes.
4. Grease container of the air fryer with cooking oil and place patties in. Air fryer at 200°C for 12 minutes.
5. Flip and air fry for an additional 8 minutes.

305. Air Fryer Polenta Chips

Total time: 55 minutes
Servings: 4

INGREDIENTS

- cup polenta
- 4- cups vegetable broth
- 4- tbsp orange juice
- oz. Parmesan cheese, grated
- Salt

INSTRUCTIONS

1. Bring vegetable stock to a boil and add in polenta, whisking till it thickens.
2. Cover and stir every 8 minutes for 45 minutes.
3. When cooked, stir in orange juice, parmesan and salt.
4. Pour polenta into a large lined tray and allow it to cool and firm up.
5. Cut into fries.
6. Preheat air fryer to 180°C.
7. Place polenta fries in air fryer basket without overlapping and spray lightly with cooking spray.
8. Cook for 15 minutes, flipping halfway through until golden brown.
9. Serve and enjoy.

306. Air Fryer Thai Salmon Patties

Total time: 25 minutes
Servings: 7

INGREDIENTS

- 400g- canned salmon

- ½- cup breadcrumbs
- 2- tsp Thai red curry paste
- 2- tsp brown sugar
- 2- eggs
- Salt and cooking spray

INSTRUCTIONS

1. Mix all the ingredients together.
2. Form 1-inch thick patties.
3. Preheat air fryer to 180°C.
4. Spray patties with cooking oil and place in air fryer basket.
5. Cook for 4 minutes on each side.

307. Air Fryer Sriracha Brussels Sprouts

Total time: 15 minutes
Servings: 3

INGREDIENTS

- 2- cups Brussels sprouts
- 1 tbsp shredded coconut
- 1 tbsp paleo sriracha
- 2 tsp sesame oil
- 2 tsp avocado oil
- Salt

INSTRUCTIONS

1. Preheat air fryer 180°C.
2. Place Brussels sprouts in a bowl and stir in sriracha, coconut and oils.
3. Toss together and coat properly.
4. Add a pinch of salt and stir.
5. Place in air fryer basket without overlapping.
6. Cook 10 to 12 minutes, shaking basket halfway through.

308. Air Fryer Nutty Chicken Tenders

Total time: 30 minutes
Servings: 4

INGREDIENTS

- 1-pound chicken tenders
- 1 egg
- ½- cup raw hazelnuts
- ½- cup raw pecan pieces
- ½- tsp garlic powder
- Salt and cooking spray

INSTRUCTIONS

1. Preheat air fryer to 180°C.
2. Cut chicken strips into 3-inch strips.
3. Whisk egg and include water, whisk once more.
4. Chop nuts in a food processor. Mix with salt and garlic powder.
5. Dip each chicken tender into the egg, then into the nut blend.
6. Spray with cooking oil and place in the air fryer bin.
7. Air fry for 12 minutes, flipping part way through.

309. Air Fryer Calzones

Total time: 27 minutes
Servings: 2

INGREDIENTS

- 3- cups baby spinach leaves
- 1/3- cup marinara sauce
- 1/3- cup shredded rotisserie chicken breast
- 6- oz. prepared whole wheat pizza dough
- 6- tsp mozzarella cheese, shredded
- Cooking spray and olive oil

INSTRUCTIONS

1. Heat oil in a sauce skillet over medium-high warm and add onion. Sauté for 2 minutes. Add spinach and butter for 2 minutes. Remove from heat and mix in marinara sauce and chicken.
2. Divide dough into 4 equivalent parts (6-inch circles).
3. Place 1/4 spinach blend into each circle. Top with cheese.
4. Fold mixture over and seal. Splash with cooking oil.
5. Place calzones in the air fryer container and cook at 160°C for 12 minutes, turning after 8 minutes.

310. Air Fryer Balsamic Tofu Bacon

Total time: 1hour 12minutes
Servings: 4

INGREDIENTS

- ¼- cup soy sauce

- 3- tbsp balsamic vinegar
- 1 tbsp maple syrup
- 1 tsp garlic powder
- 1 block firm tofu
- 1 tbsp liquid smoke

INSTRUCTIONS

1. Combine soy sauce, vinegar, maple syrup, garlic powder and liquid smoke in a bowl.
2. Place tofu in a shallow bowl and pour marinade on top.
3. Cover and marinate for 30 minutes.
4. Transfer the tofu to air fryer bin and air fry at 200°C for 18 to 23 minutes or until firm.

KETO AIR FRYER RECIPES

311. Prawn Momos

INGREDIENTS

For dough:

- 1 ½- cup all-purpose flour
- ½- tsp. salt
- 5- tbsp. water

For filling:

- 2- cups minced prawn
- 2- tbsp. oil
- 2- tsp. ginger-garlic paste
- 2- tsp. soy sauce
- 2- tsp. vinegar

INSTRUCTIONS

1. Mix the dough, cover it with saran wrap and set aside.
2. Mix the filling ingredients.
3. Fold the dough and cut it into a square.
4. Place the filling in the middle.
5. Wrap the dough to cover the filling and squeeze the edges together.
6. Preheat the Air Fryer to 200° F for 5 minutes.
7. Place in the fry bin and cook for 20 minutes.

312. Lamb fries

INGREDIENTS

- 1 lb. boneless lamb cut into fingers
- 2 cup dry breadcrumbs
- 2 tsp. oregano
- 2- tsp. red chili flakes

Marinade:

- 1 ½- tbsp. ginger-garlic paste
- 4- tbsp. lemon juice
- 2- tsp. salt
- 1 tsp. pepper powder
- 1 tsp. red chili powder
- 6- tbsp. corn flour
- 4 -eggs

INSTRUCTIONS

1. Blend all marinade ingredients and soak the meat for 20-30 minutes.
2. Blend the breadcrumbs, oregano and red chili well and dip the marinated fingers in this mix.
3. Preheat the Air Fryer to 160 F for 5 minutes.
4. Cook for 15 minutes, shaking halfway through.

313. Venison Fingers

INGREDIENTS:

- 1 lb. boneless venison cut into fingers
- 2 cup dry breadcrumbs
- 2 tsp. oregano
- 2- tsp. red chili flakes
- 2- tsp. garlic paste

Marinade:

- 1 ½- tbsp. ginger-garlic paste
- 4- tbsp. lemon juice
- 2 -tsp. salt
- 1 -tsp. red chili powder
- 6 -tbsp. corn flour
- 4 -eggs

INSTRUCTIONS

1. Blend all the marinade ingredients and soak the venison fingers for 20-30 minutes.
2. Blend the breadcrumbs, oregano and red chili well and dip the marinated fingers in this mix.
3. Preheat the Air Fryer to 160 F for 5 minutes.
4. Cook for 15 minutes, shaking halfway through.
5. Top with garlic paste and serve.

314. Cheese Chicken Fries

INGREDIENTS

- 1 lb. chicken

For the marinade:

- 1 tbsp. olive oil
- 1 tsp. mixed herbs

- ½ -tsp. red chili flakes
- A pinch of salt to taste
- 1 tbsp. lemon juice

For the garnish:

- 1 cup melted cheddar

INSTRUCTIONS

1. Mix all the marinade ingredients well
2. Cook the chicken tenders and in the marinade.
3. Preheat the Air Fryer to 300 F. Take the basket of the fryer and place the chicken strips in them.
4. Close the container. Cook for 20 or 25 minutes. Toss 2-3 times.
5. Sprinkle the cut coriander leaves on the fries.
6. Pour the melted cheese over the fries and serve hot.

315. Venison Wontons

INGREDIENTS

For dough:

- 1 ½- cup all-purpose flour
- ½- tsp. salt
- 5- tbsp. water

For filling:

- 2- cups minced venison
- 2- tbsp. oil
- 2- tsp. ginger-garlic paste
- 2- tsp. soy sauce
- 2- tsp. vinegar

INSTRUCTIONS

1. Make the dough, cover it with saran wrap and set aside.
2. Next, mix the filling ingredients.
3. Roll the batter and place the filling inside.
4. Wrap the mixture to cover the filling and squeeze the edges together.
5. Preheat the Air Fryer to 200° F for 5 minutes.
6. Place the wontons in the fry crate and cook for 20 minutes.

316. Chicken Croquette

INGREDIENTS

- 2- lb. boneless chicken

1st Marinade:

- 3- tbsp. vinegar or lemon juice
- 2 or 3 tsp. paprika
- 1 tsp. black pepper
- 1 tsp. salt
- 3 tsp. ginger-garlic paste

2nd Marinade:

- 1 cup yogurt
- 4- tsp. tandoori masala
- 2- tbsp. dry fenugreek leaves
- 1 tsp. black salt
- 1 tsp. chat masala
- 1 tsp. garam masala powder
- 1 tsp. red chili powder
- 1 tsp. salt
- 3- drops of red color

INSTRUCTIONS

1. Make the 1st marinade and drench the chicken in it for 4 hours.
2. Make the 2nd marinade and sprinkle the chicken in it to let the flavors blend.
3. Preheat the Air Fryer to 160 F and cook for 15 minutes.
4. Serve with mint chutney.

317. Veal Chili

INGREDIENTS

- 1 lb. veal
- 2 ½- tsp. ginger-garlic paste
- 1 tsp. red chili sauce
- ¼- tsp. salt
- ¼- tsp. red chili powder/black pepper
- Edible orange food coloring

For sauce:

- 2- tbsp. olive oil
- 1 ½- tsp. ginger garlic paste
- ½- tbsp. red chili sauce

- 2 -tbsp. tomato ketchup
- 2- tsp. soy sauce
- 1-2 tbsp. honey
- ¼- tsp. Ajinomoto
- 1-2 tsp. red chili flakes

INSTRUCTIONS

1. Blend all of the components for the marinade and marinate veal fingers for 30 minutes.
2. Blend the breadcrumbs, oregano and red chili flakes and add the marinated fingers on this mix.
3. Preheat the Air Fryer to 160 F and cook for 15 minutes, shaking the fry basket occasionally.

318. Pork Kebab

INGREDIENTS

- 1 lb. boneless pork cubed
- 3 -onions chopped
- 5 -green chilies-roughly chopped
- 1 ½- tbsp. ginger paste
- 1 ½ -tsp. garlic paste
- 1 ½ -tsp. salt
- 3- tsp. lemon juice
- 2 tsp. garam masala
- 4 -tbsp. chopped coriander
- 3 -tbsp. cream
- 2 -tbsp. coriander powder
- 4 -tbsp. fresh mint chopped
- 3 -tbsp. chopped capsicum
- 3 -eggs
- 2 ½ -tbsp. white sesame seeds

INSTRUCTIONS

1. Mix the pork with the ground ginger and cut green chilies.
2. Pound this blend until it turns into a thick paste.
3. Add water if required. Add the onions, mint, breadcrumbs and spices.
4. Blend this well until you get a soft mixture.
5. Form round kebabs with the dough.
6. Pour a small amount of milk onto each kebab to wet it.
7. Roll the kebab in the dry breadcrumbs.
8. Preheat the Air Fryer for 5 minutes at 300 F and cook for 30 minutes.

9. Recommended sides for this dish are mint chutney, tomato ketchup or yogurt chutney.

319. Veal patties

INGREDIENTS

- ½ -lb. minced veal
- ½ -cup breadcrumbs
- A pinch of salt to taste
- ¼ -tsp. ginger finely chopped
- 1 -green chili finely chopped
- 1 -tsp. lemon juice
- 1 -tbsp. fresh coriander leaves
- ¼ -tsp. red chili powder
- ½ -cup of boiled peas
- ¼ -tsp. cumin powder
- ¼ -tsp. dried mango powder

INSTRUCTIONS

1. Combine the ingredients. Form round cutlets with the mixture.
2. Preheat the Air Fryer to 250 F for 5 minutes and cook for 10-12 minutes.
3. Serve hot with mint chutney.

320. Pork Wontons

INGREDIENTS

For dough:

- 1 ½ -cup all-purpose flour
- ½ -tsp. salt
- 5 -tbsp. water

For filling:

- 2 -cups minced pork
- 2 -tbsp. oil
- 2 -tsp. ginger-garlic paste
- 2 -tsp. soy sauce
- 2 -tsp. vinegar

INSTRUCTIONS

1. Ply the batter and spread it with saran wrap and set aside.
2. Next, cook the elements for the filling and attempt to guarantee that the pork is secured well with the sauce.

3. Roll the batter and place the filling inside.
4. Presently, wrap the batter to cover the filling and squeeze the edges together.
5. Preheat the Air Fryer to 200° F for 5 minutes.
6. Place the wontons in the fry container and close it.
7. Give them a chance to cook at a similar temperature for an additional 20 minutes.
8. Suggested sides are stew sauce or ketchup.

321. Veal club sandwich

INGREDIENTS

- 2- slices of white bread
- 1 tbsp. softened butter
- ½- lb. cubed veal
- 1 small capsicum
- For Barbeque Sauce:
- ¼- tbsp. Worcestershire sauce
- ½- tsp. olive oil
- ½- flake garlic crushed
- ¼- cup chopped onion
- ¼- tsp. mustard powder
- ½- tbsp. sugar
- ¼- tbsp. red chili sauce
- ½- cup water

INSTRUCTIONS

1. Cut the bread diagonally.
2. Cook the sauce ingredients and until it thickens.
3. Add the veal to the sauce and mix.
4. Cook the capsicum and strip the skin off. Cut the capsicum into strips.
5. Assemble sandwich filling between bread slices.
6. Preheat the air fryer for 5 minutes at 300 F and cook for 15 minutes.

322. Chili Cheese Pork

INGREDIENTS

For pork fingers:

- 1 lb. pork
- 2 ½- tsp. ginger-garlic paste
- 1 tsp. red chili sauce
- ¼ -tsp. salt
- ¼- tsp. red chili powder/black pepper

- Edible orange food coloring

For sauce:

- 2- tbsp. olive oil
- 1 ½- tsp. ginger garlic paste
- ½ -tbsp. red chili sauce
- 2 -tbsp. tomato ketchup
- 2 -tsp. soy sauce
- 1-2 tbsp. honey
- ¼- tsp. Ajinomoto
- 1-2 tsp. red chili flakes

INSTRUCTIONS

1. Blend all of the components for the marinade and marinate veal fingers for 30 minutes.
2. Blend the breadcrumbs, oregano and red chili flakes and add the marinated fingers on this mix.
3. Preheat the Air Fryer to 160 F and cook for 15 minutes, shaking the fry basket occasionally.

323. Beef Steak fingers

INGREDIENTS

- 1 lb. boneless beef steak
- 2 cup dry breadcrumbs
- 2 tsp. oregano
- 2- tsp. red chili flakes

Marinade:

- 1 ½- tbsp. ginger-garlic paste
- 4- tbsp. lemon juice
- 2- tsp. salt
- 1 tsp. pepper powder
- 1 tsp. red chili powder
- 6- tbsp. corn flour
- 4- eggs

INSTRUCTIONS

1. Blend all marinade ingredients and soak the meat for 20-30 minutes.
2. Blend the breadcrumbs, oregano and red chili well and dip the marinated fingers in this mix.
3. Preheat the Air Fryer to 160 F for 5 minutes. Cook for 15 minutes, shaking halfway through.

324.   Fish club sandwich

INGREDIENTS

- 2- slices of white bread
- 1 -tbsp. softened butter
- 1 tin tuna
- 1 small capsicum

For Barbeque Sauce:

- ¼- tbsp. Worcestershire sauce
- ½- tsp. olive oil
- ½- flake garlic
- ¼- cup chopped onion
- ¼- tsp. mustard powder
- ½- tbsp. sugar
- ¼- tbsp. red chili sauce
- 1 tbsp. tomato ketchup
- ½- cup water.
- A pinch of salt and black pepper

INSTRUCTIONS

1. Cut the bread diagonally.
2. Cook the sauce ingredients and until it thickens.
3. Add the potato to the sauce and mix. Cook the capsicum and strip the skin off. Cut the capsicum into strips. Assemble sandwich filling between bread slices.
4. Preheat the air fryer for 5 minutes at 300 F and cook for 15 minutes.

325.   Mutton fingers

INGREDIENTS

- 1 lb. boneless mutton
- 2- cup dry breadcrumbs
- 2- tsp. oregano
- 2- tsp. red chili flakes

Marinade:

- 1 ½- tbsp. ginger-garlic paste
- 4- tbsp. lemon juice
- 2- tsp. salt
- 1 tsp. pepper powder
- 1 tsp. red chili powder
- 6- tbsp. corn flour
- 4- eggs

INSTRUCTIONS

1. Blend all marinade ingredients and soak the meat for 20-30 minutes.
2. Blend the breadcrumbs, oregano and red chili well and dip the marinated fingers in this mix.
3. Preheat the Air Fryer to 160 F for 5 minutes.
4. Cook for 15 minutes, shaking halfway through.

326.   Pork sticks

INGREDIENTS

- 1 lb. boneless pork
- 2 cup dry breadcrumbs
- 2 tsp. oregano
- 2- tsp. red chili flakes

Marinade:

- 1 ½- tbsp. ginger-garlic paste
- 4- tbsp. lemon juice
- 2- tsp. salt
- 1 tsp. pepper powder
- 1 tsp. red chili powder
- 6- tbsp. corn flour
- 4- eggs

INSTRUCTIONS

1. Blend all marinade ingredients and soak the meat for 20-30 minutes.
2. Blend the breadcrumbs, oregano and red chili well and dip the marinated fingers in this mix.
3. Preheat the Air Fryer to 160 F for 5 minutes.
4. Cook for 15 minutes, shaking halfway through.

327.   Kyinkyinga

INGREDIENTS

- 1 -lb. boneless beef liver
- 3 -onions chopped
- 5 -green chilies-roughly
- 1 ½- tbsp. ginger paste
- 1 ½- tsp. garlic paste
- 1 ½- tsp. salt
- 3- tsp. lemon juice
- 2 tsp. garam masala
- 4- tbsp. chopped coriander
- 3- tbsp. cream
- 2 tbsp. coriander powder

- 4 tbsp. fresh mint
- 3- tbsp. chopped capsicum
- 2 tbsp. peanut flour
- 3- eggs

INSTRUCTIONS

1. Manipulate the batter and spread it with cling wrap and set aside.
2. Next, cook the elements for the filling and attempt to guarantee that the hamburger is secured well with the sauce.
3. Roll the batter and place the filling in the inside.
4. Presently, wrap the mixture to cover the filling and squeeze the edges together.
5. preheat the Air Fryer to 200° F for 5 minutes.
6. Place the wontons in the fry bin and close it.
7. Give them a chance to cook at a similar temperature for an additional 20 minutes.
8. Prescribed sides are chili sauce or ketchup.

328.   Beef Wontons

INGREDIENTS

For dough:

- 1 ½- cup all-purpose flour
- ½ -tsp. salt
- 5- tbsp. water

For filling:

- 2- cups minced beef steak
- 2- tbsp. oil
- 2- tsp. ginger-garlic paste
- 2- tsp. soy sauce
- 2- tsp. vinegar

INSTRUCTIONS

1. Ply the batter and spread it with saran wrap and set aside.
2. Next, cook the elements for the filling and attempt to guarantee that the pork is secured well with the sauce.
3. Roll the batter and place the filling inside.
4. Presently, wrap the batter to cover the filling and squeeze the edges together.
5. Preheat the Air Fryer to 200° F for 5 minutes.

6. Place the wontons in the fry container and close it.
7. Give them a chance to cook at a similar temperature for an additional 20 minutes.
8. Suggested sides are stew sauce or ketchup.

329.   Prawn Samosa

INGREDIENTS

For wrappers:

- 2- tbsp. unsalted butter
- 1 ½- cup all-purpose flour
- A pinch of salt to taste
- Add as much water as required

For filling:

- 1 lb. prawn
- ¼- cup boiled peas
- 1 -tsp. powdered ginger
- 1 or 2 green chilies
- ½- tsp. cumin
- 1 tsp. coarsely crushed coriander
- 1 dry red chili broken into pieces
- A small amount of salt
- ½- tsp. dried mango powder
- ½- tsp. red chili powder.
- 1-2- tbsp. coriander.

INSTRUCTIONS

1. Blend the wrapper ingredients. Let it sit while making the filling.
2. Cook the ingredients in a skillet and blend them well to make a thick paste.
3. Form the paste into balls. Cut them in half and insert the filling.
4. Preheat the Air Fryer to 300 F. Place the samosas in the fry receptacle.
5. Cook for 20-25 minutes. Flip halfway through for uniform cooking.
6. Serve hot with tamarind or mint chutney.

330. Juicy Chicken Kebab

INGREDIENTS

- 2 lb. chicken breasts cubed
- 3 onions chopped
- 5- green chilies-roughly chopped
- 1 ½- tbsp. ginger paste
- 1 ½- tsp. garlic paste
- 1 ½- tsp. salt
- 3- tsp. lemon juice
- 2 tsp. garam masala
- 4- tbsp. chopped coriander
- 3- tbsp. cream
- 2 tbsp. coriander powder
- 4- tbsp. fresh mint (chopped)
- 3- tbsp. chopped capsicum
- 2 tbsp. peanut flour
- 3- eggs

INSTRUCTIONS

1. Mix the chicken with the ground ginger and cut green chilies.
2. Pound this blend until it turns into a thick paste.
3. Add water if required. Add the onions, mint, breadcrumbs and spices.
4. Blend this well until you get a soft mixture.
5. Form round kebabs with the dough.
6. Pour a small amount of milk onto each kebab to wet it.
7. Roll the kebab in the dry breadcrumbs.
8. Preheat the Air Fryer for 5 minutes at 300 F and cook for 30 minutes.
9. Recommended sides for this dish are mint chutney, tomato ketchup or yogurt chutney.

331. Chicken Momos

INGREDIENTS

For dough:

- 1 ½- cup all-purpose flour
- ½- tsp. salt
- 5- tbsp. water

For filling:

- 2- cups minced chicken
- 2- tbsp. oil
- 2- tsp. ginger-garlic paste
- 2- tsp. soy sauce
- 2- tsp. vinegar

INSTRUCTIONS

1. Mix the dough, cover it with saran wrap and set aside.
2. Mix the filling ingredients.
3. Fold the dough and cut it into a square. Place the filling in the middle. Wrap the dough to cover the filling and squeeze the edges together.
4. Preheat the Air Fryer to 200° F for 5 minutes. Place in the fry bin and cook for 20 minutes.

332. Lamb Momos

INGREDIENTS

For dough:

- 1 ½- cup all-purpose flour
- ½- tsp. salt
- 5- tbsp. water

For filling:

- 2- cups minced lamb
- 2- tbsp. oil
- 2- tsp. ginger-garlic paste
- 2- tsp. soy sauce
- 2- tsp. vinegar

INSTRUCTIONS

1. Mix the dough, cover it with saran wrap and set aside.
2. Mix the filling ingredients.
3. Fold the dough and cut it into a square.
4. Place the filling in the middle.
5. Wrap the dough to cover the filling and squeeze the edges together.
6. Preheat the Air Fryer to 200° F for 5 minutes. Place in the fry bin and cook for 20 minutes.

333. Beef steak Momos

INGREDIENTS

For dough:

- 1 ½- cup all-purpose flour

- ½- tsp. salt
- 5 -tbsp. water

For filling:

- 2- cups minced beef steak
- 2- tbsp. oil
- 2- tsp. ginger-garlic paste
- 2- tsp. soy sauce
- 2- tsp. vinegar

INSTRUCTIONS

1. Mix the dough, cover it with saran wrap and set aside.
2. Mix the filling ingredients.
3. Fold the dough and cut it into a square.
4. Place the filling in the middle.
5. Wrap the dough to cover the filling and squeeze the edges together.
6. Preheat the Air Fryer to 200° F for 5 minutes.
7. Place in the fry bin and cook for 20 minutes.

334. Chicken Tikka

INGREDIENTS

- 2- cups sliced chicken
- 1 large capsicum
- 1 onion
- 5- tbsp. gram flour
- A pinch of salt to taste
- For the filling:
- 2 cup fresh green coriander
- ½- cup mint leaves
- 4- tsp. fennel
- 2 tbsp. ginger-garlic paste
- 1 small onion
- 6-7 flakes garlic
- Salt
- 3- tbsp. lemon juice

INSTRUCTIONS

1. You will first need to make the chutney.
2. Add the ingredients to a blender and make a thick paste.
3. Cut the bits of chicken and stuff a large segment of the paste into the pit procured.
4. Take the remainder of the paste and add it to the gram flour and salt.

5. Heave the bits of chicken in this mix and put it in a protected place.
6. Apply a smidgen of the mix on the capsicum and onion.
7. Recognize these on a stick close by the chicken pieces.
8. Preheat the Air Fryer to 290 F for around 5 minutes.
9. Open the holder. Coordinate the satay sticks suitably.
10. Close the basket.
11. Keep the sticks with the chicken at 180 for around thirty minutes while the sticks with the vegetables are to be kept at a comparable temperature for only 7 minutes.
12. Turn the sticks in with the objective that one side doesn't get burned and moreover to give a uniform cooking.

335. Pork Tandoor

INGREDIENTS

- 2- cups sliced pork belly
- 1 large capsicum
- 1 onion
- 5- tbsp. gram flour
- A pinch of salt to taste
- For the filling:
- 2 cup fresh green coriander
- ½- cup mint leaves
- 4- tsp. fennel
- 2 tbsp. ginger-garlic paste
- 1 small onion
- 6-7 flakes garlic
- Salt
- 3- tbsp. lemon juice

INSTRUCTIONS

1. You will first need to make the chutney.
2. Add the ingredients to a blender and make a thick paste.
3. Cut the bits of pork and stuff a large bit of the paste into space got.
4. Take the remainder of the paste and add it to the gram flour and salt.
5. Throw the bits of Pork on this blend and positioned it in a covered place.
6. Apply a hint of the mixture at the capsicum and onion.

7. Recognize those on a stick close by the red meat portions.
8. Preheat the Air Fryer to 290 F for around 5 minutes.
9. Keep the sticks with the beef at 180 levels for around thirty minutes even as the sticks with the greens are to be stored at a similar temperature for best 7 minutes.
10. Turn the sticks in with the goal that one facet would not get seared and except to provide a uniform cooking.

336. Mutton Tikka

INGREDIENTS

- 2- cups sliced mutton
- 1 large capsicum
- 1 onion
- 5- tbsp. gram flour
- A pinch of salt to taste

For the filling:

- 2- cup fresh green coriander
- ½- cup mint leaves
- 4- tsp. fennel
- 2 tbsp. ginger-garlic paste
- 1 small onion
- 6-7 flakes garlic
- Salt
- 3- tbsp. lemon juice

INSTRUCTIONS

1. You will initially want to make the chutney.
2. Add the substances to a blender and make a thick paste.
3. Cut the bits of sheep and stuff a large portion of the paste into the cavity got.
4. Take the relaxation of the paste and upload it to the gram flour and salt.
5. Toss the bits of sheep on this blend and put it in a safe place.
6. Apply a smidgen of the blend at the capsicum and onion.
7. Place those on a stick along with the lamb pieces.
8. Preheat the Air Fryer to 290 F for around 5 minutes.
9. Open the bin. Arrange the stay sticks as they should be.

10. Close the crate. Keep the sticks with the mutton at 180 ranges for around half an hour while the sticks with the vegetables are to be stored on the identical temperature for only 7 minutes.
11. Turn the sticks in between so that one facet does no longer get burnt and additionally to offer a uniform cook dinner.

337. Chicken Wontons

INGREDIENTS

For dough:

- 1 ½- cup all-purpose flour
- ½- tsp. salt
- 5- tbsp. water

For filling:

- 2- cups minced chicken
- 2- tbsp. oil
- 2- tsp. ginger-garlic paste
- 2- tsp. soy sauce
- 2- tsp. vinegar

INSTRUCTIONS

1. Mix the dough, cover it with saran wrap and set aside.
2. Mix the filling ingredients.
3. Fold the dough and cut it into a square.
4. Place the filling in the middle.
5. Wrap the dough to cover the filling and squeeze the edges together.
6. Preheat the Air Fryer to 200° F for 5 minutes.
7. Place in the fry bin and cook for 20 minutes.

338. Beef Steak

INGREDIENTS

- 2- lb. boneless beef cut into slices

1st Marinade:

- 3- tbsp. vinegar or lemon juice
- 2 or 3 tsp. paprika
- 1 tsp. black pepper
- 1 tsp. salt
- 3 tsp. ginger-garlic paste

2nd Marinade:

- 1 cup yogurt
- 4- tsp. tandoori masala
- 2 tbsp. dry fenugreek leaves
- 1 tsp. black salt
- 1 tsp. chat masala
- 1 tsp. garam masala powder
- 1 tsp. red chili powder
- 1 tsp. salt
- 3- drops of red color

INSTRUCTIONS

1. Make the first marinade and soak the cut pork in it for 4 hours.
2. While that is occurring, make the second one marinade and soak the pork in it overnight to allow the flavors to combine.
3. Preheat the Air Fryer to 10060 ranges F for 5 minutes.
4. Place the fingers inside the fry basket and near it.
5. Let them prepare dinner at the same temperature for another 15 minutes or so.
6. Toss the arms nicely so that they're cooked uniformly.
7. Serve them with mint chutney.

339.   Chicken Samosa

INGREDIENTS

For wrappers:

- 2 tbsp. unsalted butter
- 1 ½- cup all-purpose flour
- A pinch of salt to taste
- Add as much water as required

For filling:

- 1 lb. chicken
- ¼- cup boiled peas
- 1 tsp. powdered ginger
- 1 or 2 green chilies
- ½- tsp. cumin
- 1 tsp. coarsely crushed coriander
- 1 dry red chili broken into pieces
- A small amount of salt (to taste)
- ½- tsp. dried mango powder
- ½- tsp. red chili powder.

- 1-2 tbsp. coriander.

INSTRUCTIONS

1. Blend the wrapper ingredients. Let it sit while making the filling.
2. Cook the ingredients in a skillet and blend them well to make a thick paste.
3. Form the paste into balls. Cut them in half and insert the filling.
4. Preheat the Air Fryer to 300 F. Place the samosas in the fry receptacle.
5. Cook for 20-25 minutes. Flip halfway through for uniform cooking.
6. Serve hot with tamarind or mint chutney.

340.   Fish Kebab

INGREDIENTS

- 1 -lb. boneless fish
- 3- onions chopped
- 5- green chilies-roughly chopped
- 1 ½- tbsp. ginger paste
- 1 ½- tsp garlic paste
- 1 ½- tsp salt
- 3- tsp lemon juice
- 2 tsp garam masala
- 4- tbsp. chopped coriander
- 3- tbsp. cream
- 2 tbsp. coriander powder
- 4- tbsp. fresh mint chopped
- 3- tbsp. chopped capsicum
- 3- eggs
- 2 ½- tbsp. white sesame seeds

INSTRUCTIONS

1. Mix the fish with the ground ginger and cut green chilies.
2. Pound this blend until it turns into a thick paste. Add water if required.
3. Add the onions, mint, breadcrumbs and spices.
4. Blend this well until you get a soft mixture.
5. Form round kebabs with the dough.
6. Pour a small amount of milk onto each kebab to wet it.
7. Roll the kebab in the dry breadcrumbs.
8. Preheat the Air Fryer for 5 minutes at 300 F and cook for 30 minutes.

9. Recommended sides for this dish are mint chutney, tomato ketchup or yogurt chutney.

341. Fish fingers

INGREDIENTS

- ½- lb. firm white fish fillet
- 1 tbsp. lemon juice
- 2 cups of dry breadcrumbs
- 1 cup oil for frying

Marinade:

- 1 ½- tbsp. ginger-garlic paste
- 3- tbsp. lemon juice
- 2 tsp salt
- 1 ½- tsp pepper powder
- 1 tsp red chili flakes or to taste
- 3 eggs
- 5 tbsp. corn flour
- 2 tsp tomato ketchup

INSTRUCTIONS

1. Blend all marinade ingredients and soak the meat for 20-30 minutes.
2. Blend the breadcrumbs, oregano and red chili well and dip the marinated fingers in this mix.
3. Preheat the Air Fryer to 160 F for 5 minutes.
4. Cook for 15 minutes, shaking halfway through.

342. Chinese Chili

INGREDIENTS

For chicken fingers:

- 1 lb. chicken
- 2 ½- tsp. ginger-garlic paste
- 1 tsp. red chili sauce
- ¼- tsp. salt
- ¼- tsp. red chili powder/black pepper
- Edible orange food coloring

For sauce:

- 2- tbsp. olive oil
- 1 ½- tsp. ginger garlic paste
- ½- tbsp. red chili sauce
- 2- tbsp. tomato ketchup
- 2- tsp. soy sauce

- 1-2- tbsp. honey
- ¼- tsp. Ajinomoto
- 1-2- tsp. red chili flakes

INSTRUCTIONS

1. Blend all of the components for the marinade and marinate chicken fingers for 30 minutes.
2. Blend the breadcrumbs, oregano and red chili flakes and add the marinated fingers on this mix.
3. Preheat the Air Fryer to 160 F and cook for 15 minutes, shaking the fry basket occasionally.

343. Lamb Kebab

INGREDIENTS

- 1 lb. of lamb
- 3- onions chopped
- 5- green chilies-roughly chopped
- 1 ½- tbsp. ginger paste
- 1 ½- tsp garlic paste
- 1 ½- tsp salt
- 3 tsp lemon juice
- 2 tsp garam masala
- 4 tbsp. chopped coriander
- 3 tbsp. cream
- 4 tbsp. fresh mint chopped
- 3 tbsp. chopped capsicum
- 3 eggs
- 2 ½- tbsp. white sesame seeds

INSTRUCTIONS

1. Mix the lamb with the ground ginger and cut green chilies.
2. Pound this blend until it turns into a thick paste. Add water if required.
3. Add the onions, mint, breadcrumbs and spices.
4. Blend this well until you get a soft mixture.
5. Form round kebabs with the dough.
6. Pour a small amount of milk onto each kebab to wet it.
7. Roll the kebab in the dry breadcrumbs.
8. Preheat the Air Fryer for 5 minutes at 300 F and cook for 30 minutes.
9. Recommended sides for this dish are mint chutney, tomato ketchup or yogurt chutney.

344. Mutton Samosas

INGREDIENTS

For wrappers:

- 2- tbsp. unsalted butter
- 1 ½- cup all-purpose flour
- A pinch of salt to taste
- Add as much water as required

For filling:

- 2 cups minced mutton
- ¼- cup boiled peas
- A small amount of ginger
- 1 or 2 green chilies
- ½ -tsp cumin
- 1 tsp coarsely crushed coriander
- 1 dry red chili broken into pieces
- A small amount of salt
- ½- tsp dried mango powder
- ½- tsp red chili powder
- 1-2 tbsp. coriander

INSTRUCTIONS

1. Blend the wrapper ingredients. Let it sit while making the filling.
2. Cook the ingredients in a skillet and blend them well to make a thick paste.
3. Form the paste into balls. Cut them in half and insert the filling.
4. Preheat the Air Fryer to 300 F. Place the samosas in the fry receptacle.
5. Cook for 20-25 minutes. Flip halfway through for uniform cooking.
6. Serve hot with tamarind or mint chutney.

345. Prawn Wontons

INGREDIENTS

For dough:

- 1 ½- cup all-purpose flour
- ½- tsp. salt
- 5- tbsp. water

For filling:

- 2- cups minced prawn

- 2- tbsp. oil
- 2- tsp. ginger-garlic paste
- 2- tsp. soy sauce
- 2- tsp. vinegar

INSTRUCTIONS

1. Mix the dough, cover it with saran wrap and set aside.
2. Mix the filling ingredients.
3. Fold the dough and cut it into a square.
4. Place the filling in the middle.
5. Wrap the dough to cover the filling and squeeze the edges together.
6. Preheat the Air Fryer to 200° F for 5 minutes.
7. Place in the fry bin and cook for 20 minutes.

346. Lamb Club Sandwich

INGREDIENTS

- 2 slices of white bread
- 1 tbsp. softened butter
- ½- lb. cut lamb
- 1 small capsicum

Barbeque Sauce:

- ¼- tbsp. Worcestershire sauce
- ½- tsp. olive oil
- ½- flake garlic crushed
- ¼- cup chopped onion
- ½- tbsp. sugar
- ¼- tbsp. red chili sauce

INSTRUCTIONS

1. Cut the bread diagonally.
2. Cook the sauce ingredients and until it thickens.
3. Add the lamb to the sauce and mix. Cook the capsicum and strip the skin off.
4. Cut the capsicum into strips. Assemble sandwich filling between bread slices.
5. Preheat the air fryer for 5 minutes at 300 F and cook for 15 minutes.

347. Honey Chili Chicken

INGREDIENTS

For chicken fingers:

- 1 lb. chicken
- 2 ½- tsp. ginger-garlic paste
- 1 tsp. red chili sauce
- ¼- tsp. salt
- ¼- tsp. red chili powder
- Edible orange food coloring

For sauce:

- 2 tbsp. olive oil
- 1 capsicum
- 2 small onions
- 1 ½- tsp. ginger garlic paste
- ½- tbsp. red chili sauce
- 2 tbsp. tomato ketchup
- 1 ½- tbsp. sweet chili sauce
- 2 tsp. soy sauce
- 2 tsp. vinegar
- 1-2 tbsp. honey
- A pinch of black pepper
- 2 tsp. red chili flakes

INSTRUCTIONS

1. Blend all of the components for the marinade and marinate veal fingers for 30 minutes.
2. Blend the breadcrumbs, oregano and red chili flakes and add the marinated fingers on this mix.
3. Preheat the Air Fryer to 160 F and cook for 15 minutes, shaking the fry basket occasionally.

348. Beef Samosa

INGREDIENTS

For wrappers:

- 2 tbsp. unsalted butter
- 1 ½- cup all-purpose flour
- A pinch of salt
- Add as much water as required

For filling:

- 2 cups minced beef

- ¼- cup boiled peas
- 1 or 2- green chilies
- ½ -tsp cumin
- 1 tsp coarsely crushed whole coriander
- 1 -dry red chili
- A small amount of salt
- 1 tsp. coriander seeds

INSTRUCTIONS

1. Blend the wrapper ingredients. Let it sit while making the filling.
2. Cook the ingredients in a skillet and blend them well to make a thick paste.
3. Form the paste into balls. Cut them in half and insert the filling.
4. Preheat the Air Fryer to 300 F. Place the samosas in the fry receptacle.
5. Cook for 20-25 minutes. Flip halfway through for uniform cooking.
6. Serve hot with tamarind or mint chutney.

349. Veal Momos

INGREDIENTS

For dough:

- 1 ½- cup all-purpose flour
- ½- tsp. salt
- 5 -tbsp. water

For filling:

- 2 cups minced veal
- 2 tbsp. oil
- 2 tsp. ginger-garlic paste
- 2 tsp. soy sauce
- 2 tsp. vinegar

INSTRUCTIONS

1. Mix the dough, cover it with saran wrap and set aside.
2. Mix the filling ingredients.
3. Fold the dough and cut it into a square.
4. Place the filling in the middle. Wrap the dough to cover the filling and squeeze the edges together.
5. Preheat the Air Fryer to 200° F for 5 minutes.
6. Place in the fry bin and cook for 20 minutes.

350. Turkey Wontons

INGREDIENTS

For dough:

- 1 ½- cup all-purpose flour
- ½- tsp. salt
- 5- tbsp. water

For filling:

- 2- cups minced turkey
- 2- tbsp. oil
- 2- tsp. ginger-garlic paste
- 2- tsp. soy sauce
- 2- tsp. vinegar

INSTRUCTIONS

1. Mix the dough, cover it with saran wrap and set aside.
2. Mix the filling ingredients.
3. Fold the dough and cut it into a square. Place the filling in the middle.
4. Wrap the dough to cover the filling and squeeze the edges together.
5. Preheat the Air Fryer to 200° F for 5 minutes. Place in the fry bin and cook for 20 minutes.

351. Salmon Tandoor

INGREDIENTS

2 lb. boneless salmon filets

1st Marinade:

- 3 tbsp. vinegar or lemon juice
- 2 or 3 tsp. paprika
- 1 tsp. black pepper
- 1 tsp. salt
- 3 tsp. ginger-garlic paste

2nd Marinade:

- 1 cup yogurt
- 4- tsp. tandoori masala
- 2- tbsp. dry fenugreek leaves
- 1 tsp. black salt
- 1 tsp. chat masala
- 1 tsp. garam masala powder
- 1 tsp. red chili powder
- 1 tsp. salt
- 3- drops of red color

INSTRUCTIONS

1. Make the 1st marinade and drench the salmon in it for 4 hours.
2. Make the 2nd marinade and sprinkle the salmon in it to let the flavors blend.
3. Preheat the Air Fryer to 160 F and cook for 15 minutes.
4. Serve with mint chutney.

352. Quail Samosas

INGREDIENTS

For wrappers:

- 2 tbsp. unsalted butter
- 1 ½- cup all-purpose flour
- A pinch of salt to taste
- Add as much water as required

For filling:

- 1 lb. quail
- ¼- cup boiled peas
- 1 tsp. powdered ginger
- 1 or 2 green chilies
- ½- tsp. cumin
- 1 tsp. coarsely crushed coriander
- 1 dry red chili broken into pieces
- A small amount of salt
- ½- tsp. dried mango powder
- ½- tsp. red chili power.
- 1-2- tbsp. coriander.

INSTRUCTIONS

1. Blend the wrapper ingredients. Let it sit while making the filling.
2. Cook the ingredients in a skillet and blend them well to make a thick paste.
3. Form the paste into balls. Cut them in half and insert the filling.
4. Preheat the Air Fryer to 300 F. Place the samosas in the fry receptacle.
5. Cook for 20-25 minutes. Flip halfway through for uniform cooking.
6. Serve hot with tamarind or mint chutney.

353. Turkey Burger Cutlets

INGREDIENTS

- ½- lb. minced turkey
- ½- cup breadcrumbs
- A pinch of salt
- ¼- tsp. ginger
- 1 green chili
- 1 tsp. lemon juice
- 1 tbsp. fresh coriander leaves.
- ¼- tsp. red chili powder
- ½- cup of boiled peas
- ¼- tsp. cumin powder
- ¼- tsp. dried mango powder

INSTRUCTIONS

1. Combine the ingredients. Form round cutlets with the mixture.
2. Preheat the Air Fryer to 250 F for 5 minutes and cook for 10-12 minutes.
3. Serve hot with mint chutney.

354. Shrimp Momos

INGREDIENTS

For dough:

- 1 ½- cup all-purpose flour
- ½- tsp. salt
- 5- tbsp. water

For filling:

- 2- cups minced shrimp
- 2- tbsp. oil
- 2- tsp. ginger-garlic paste
- 2- tsp. soy sauce
- 2- tsp. vinegar

INSTRUCTIONS

1. Mix the dough, cover it with saran wrap and set aside.
2. Mix the filling ingredients.
3. Fold the dough and cut it into a square. Place the filling in the middle.
4. Wrap the dough to cover the filling and squeeze the edges together.
5. Preheat the Air Fryer to 200° F for 5 minutes.

6. Place in the fry bin and cook for 20 minutes.

355. Salmon fries

INGREDIENTS

- 1 lb. boneless salmon filets
- 2 cup dry breadcrumbs
- 2 tsp. oregano
- 2 tsp. red chili flakes

Marinade:

- 1 ½- tbsp. ginger-garlic paste
- 4 tbsp. lemon juice
- 2 tsp. salt
- 1 tsp. pepper powder
- 1 tsp. red chili powder
- 6- tbsp. corn flour
- 4- eggs

INSTRUCTIONS

1. Blend all marinade ingredients and soak the meat for 20-30 minutes.
2. Blend the breadcrumbs, oregano and red chili well and dip the marinated fingers in this mix.
3. Preheat the Air Fryer to 160 F for 5 minutes.
4. Cook for 15 minutes, shaking halfway through.

356. Oyster Club Sandwich

INGREDIENTS

- 2 slices of white bread
- 1 tbsp. softened butter
- ½- lb. shelled oyster
- 1 small capsicum

For Barbeque Sauce:

- ¼- tbsp. Worcestershire sauce
- ½- tsp. olive oil
- ½- flake garlic crushed
- ¼- cup chopped onion
- ¼- tsp. mustard powder
- 1 tbsp. tomato ketchup
- ½- tbsp. sugar
- ¼- tbsp. red chili sauce
- ½- cup water.
- A pinch of salt and black pepper

INSTRUCTIONS

1. Cut the bread diagonally.
2. Cook the sauce ingredients and until it thickens.
3. Add the oyster to the sauce and mix. Cook the capsicum and strip the skin off.
4. Cut the capsicum into strips. Assemble sandwich filling between bread slices.
5. Preheat the air fryer for 5 minutes at 300 F and cook for 15 minutes.
6. Serve the sandwiches with tomato ketchup or mint chutney.

357. Quail Chili

INGREDIENTS

- 1 lb. quail
- 2 ½- tsp. ginger-garlic paste
- 1 tsp. red chili sauce
- ¼- tsp. salt
- ¼- tsp. red chili powder/black pepper
- Edible orange food coloring

For sauce:

- 2 tbsp. olive oil
- 1 ½- tsp. ginger garlic paste
- ½- tbsp. red chili sauce
- 2 tbsp. tomato ketchup
- 2 tsp. soy sauce
- 1-2- tbsp. honey
- ¼- tsp. Ajinomoto
- 1-2- tsp. red chili flakes

INSTRUCTIONS

1. Blend all of the components for the marinade and marinate veal fingers for 30 minutes.
2. Blend the breadcrumbs, oregano and red chili flakes and add the marinated fingers on this mix.
3. Preheat the Air Fryer to 160 F and cook for 15 minutes, shaking the fry basket occasionally.

358. Cheese Carp Fries

INGREDIENTS

- 1 lb. carp fingers
- Ingredients: for the marinade:

- 1 tbsp. olive oil
- 1 tsp. mixed herbs
- ½- tsp. red chili flakes
- A pinch of salt to taste
- 1 tbsp. lemon juice

For the garnish:

- 1 cup melted cheddar

INSTRUCTIONS

1. Blend all marinade ingredients and soak the meat for 20-30 minutes.
2. Blend the breadcrumbs, oregano and red chili well and dip the marinated fingers in this mix.
3. Preheat the Air Fryer to 160 F for 5 minutes. Cook for 15 minutes, shaking halfway through.

359. Duck fingers

INGREDIENTS

- 1 lb. boneless duck
- 2 cup dry breadcrumbs
- 2 tsp. oregano
- 2 tsp. red chili flakes

Marinade:

- 1 ½- tbsp. ginger-garlic paste
- 4- tbsp. lemon juice
- 2 tsp. salt
- 1 tsp. pepper powder
- 1 tsp. red chili powder
- 6- tbsp. corn flour
- 4- eggs

INSTRUCTIONS

1. Blend all marinade ingredients and soak the meat for 20-30 minutes.
2. Blend the breadcrumbs, oregano and red chili well and dip the marinated fingers in this mix.
3. Preheat the Air Fryer to 160 F for 5 minutes. Cook for 15 minutes, shaking halfway through.

360.   Lobster Wontons

INGREDIENTS

For dough:

- 1 ½- cup all-purpose flour
- ½- tsp. salt
- 5- tbsp. water

For filling:

- 2- cups minced lobster
- 2- tbsp. oil
- 2- tsp. ginger-garlic paste
- 2- tsp. soy sauce
- 2- tsp. vinegar

INSTRUCTIONS

1. Mix the dough, cover it with saran wrap and set aside.
2. Mix the filling ingredients.
3. Fold the dough and cut it into a square.
4. Place the filling in the middle.
5. Wrap the dough to cover the filling and squeeze the edges together.
6. Preheat the Air Fryer to 200° F for 5 minutes. Place in the fry bin and cook for 20 minutes.

361.   Seafood Platter

INGREDIENTS

1 large plate with assorted prepared seafood

1st Marinade:

- 3- tbsp. vinegar or lemon juice
- 2 or 3- tsp. paprika
- 1 tsp. black pepper
- 1 tsp. salt
- 3- tsp. ginger-garlic paste

2nd Marinade:

- 1 cup yogurt
- 4- tsp. tandoori masala
- 2 tbsp. dry fenugreek leaves
- 1 tsp. black salt
- 1 tsp. chat masala
- 1 tsp. garam masala powder

- 1 tsp. red chili powder
- 1 tsp. salt
- 3- drops of red color

INSTRUCTIONS

1. Make the 1st marinade and drench the chicken in it for 4 hours.
2. Make the 2nd marinade and sprinkle the chicken in it to let the flavors blend.
3. Preheat the Air Fryer to 160 F and cook for 15 minutes.
4. Serve with mint chutney.

362.   Calamari Chili

INGREDIENTS

- 1 lb. calamari
- 2 ½- tsp. ginger-garlic paste
- 1 tsp. red chili sauce
- ¼- tsp. salt
- ¼- tsp. red chili powder
- Edible orange food coloring

For sauce:

- 2 tbsp. olive oil
- 1 ½- tsp. ginger garlic paste
- ½- tbsp. red chili sauce
- 2 tbsp. tomato ketchup
- 2 tsp. soy sauce
- 1-2- tbsp. honey
- ¼- tsp. Ajinomoto
- 1-2- tsp. red chili flakes

INSTRUCTIONS

1. Blend all of the components for the marinade and marinate veal fingers for 30 minutes.
2. Blend the breadcrumbs, oregano and red chili flakes and add the marinated fingers on this mix.
3. Preheat the Air Fryer to 160 F and cook for 15 minutes, shaking the fry basket occasionally.

363.   Chicken galette

INGREDIENTS

- 2 tbsp. garam masala
- 1 lb. minced chicken

- 3- tsp ginger finely chopped
- 1-2- tbsp. fresh coriander leaves
- 2 or 3- green chilies
- 1 ½- tbsp. lemon juice
- Salt and pepper

INSTRUCTIONS

1. Blend the ingredients in a bowl.
2. Form this blend into round, flat galettes.
3. Wet the galettes with a small amount of water. Coat each galette with crushed peanuts.
4. Preheat the Air Fryer to 160 F for 5 minutes.
5. Place the galettes in the fry bin and let them cook for an additional 25 minutes.
6. Continue turning them over to cook uniformly.
7. Serve with mint chutney or ketchup.

364. Mutton galette

INGREDIENTS

- 2 tbsp. garam masala
- 1 lb. minced mutton
- 3 tsp ginger finely chopped
- 1-2- tbsp. fresh coriander leaves
- 2 or 3- green chilies
- 1 ½- tbsp. lemon juice
- Salt and pepper

INSTRUCTIONS

1. Blend the ingredients in a bowl.
2. Form this blend into round, flat galettes.
3. Wet the galettes with a small amount of water. Coat each galette with crushed peanuts.
4. Preheat the Air Fryer to 160 F for 5 minutes.
5. Place the galettes in the fry bin and let them cook for an additional 25 minutes.
6. Continue turning them over to cook uniformly.
7. Serve with mint chutney or ketchup.

365. Salmon Fritters

INGREDIENTS

- 2 tbsp. garam masala
- 1 lb. fileted Salmon
- 3- tsp ginger finely chopped
- 1-2- tbsp. fresh coriander leaves

- 2 or 3- green chilies
- 1 ½- tbsp. lemon juice
- Salt and pepper to taste

INSTRUCTIONS

1. Blend the ingredients in a bowl.
2. Form this blend into round, flat galettes.
3. Wet the galettes with a small amount of water. Coat each galette with crushed peanuts.
4. Preheat the Air Fryer to 160 F for 5 minutes.
5. Place the galettes in the fry bin and let them cook for an additional 25 minutes.
6. Continue turning them over to cook uniformly.
7. Serve with mint chutney or ketchup.

366. Turkey fritters

INGREDIENTS

- 2 tbsp. garam masala
- 1 lb. minced turkey
- 3 tsp ginger finely chopped
- 1-2- tbsp. fresh coriander leaves
- 2 or 3- green chilies
- 1 ½- tbsp. lemon juice
- Salt and pepper

INSTRUCTIONS

1. Blend the ingredients in a bowl.
2. Form this blend into round, flat galettes.
3. Wet the galettes with a small amount of water. Coat each galette with crushed peanuts.
4. Preheat the Air Fryer to 160 F for 5 minutes.
5. Place the galettes in the fry bin and let them cook for an additional 25 minutes.
6. Continue turning them over to cook uniformly.
7. Serve with mint chutney or ketchup.

367. Pork Fritters

INGREDIENTS

- 2 tbsp. garam masala
- 1 lb. sliced pork
- 3 -tsp ginger finely chopped
- 1-2- tbsp. fresh coriander leaves
- 2 or 3 -green chilies
- 1 ½- tbsp. lemon juice

- Salt and pepper to taste

INSTRUCTIONS

1. Blend the ingredients in a bowl.
2. Form this blend into round, flat galettes.
3. Wet the galettes with a small amount of water. Coat each galette with crushed peanuts.
4. Preheat the Air Fryer to 160 F for 5 minutes.
5. Place the galettes in the fry bin and let them cook for an additional 25 minutes.
6. Continue turning them over to cook uniformly.
7. Serve with mint chutney or ketchup.

368. Beef Pancakes

INGREDIENTS

- 2 -tbsp. garam masala
- 1 -lb. sliced beef steak
- 3 -tsp ginger finely chopped
- 1-2 -tbsp. fresh coriander leaves
- 2 or 3- green chilies
- 1 ½ -tbsp. lemon juice
- Salt and pepper

INSTRUCTIONS

1. Blend the ingredients in a bowl and add water to it.
2. Preheat the Air Fryer to 160 F and cook for 25 minutes.
3. Continue turning them over to cook uniformly.
4. Serve either with mint chutney or ketchup.

369. Carp Pancakes

INGREDIENTS

- 2 -tbsp. garam masala
- 1 -lb. fileted carp
- 3 -tsp ginger finely chopped
- 1-2 -tbsp. fresh coriander leaves
- 2 or 3- green chilies
- 1 ½- tbsp. lemon juice
- Salt and pepper

INSTRUCTIONS

1. Blend the ingredients in a bowl and add water to it.
2. Preheat the Air Fryer to 160 F and cook for 25 minutes.
3. Continue turning them over to cook uniformly.
4. Serve either with mint chutney or ketchup.

370. Prawn galette

INGREDIENTS

- 2 tbsp. garam masala
- 1 lb. minced prawn
- 3- tsp ginger finely chopped
- 1-2- tbsp. fresh coriander leaves
- 2 or 3- green chilies
- 1 ½- tbsp. lemon juice
- Salt and pepper

INSTRUCTIONS

1. Blend the ingredients in a bowl.
2. Form this blend into round, flat galettes.
3. Wet the galettes with a small amount of water. Coat each galette with crushed peanuts.
4. Preheat the Air Fryer to 160 F for 5 minutes.
5. Place the galettes in the fry bin and let them cook for an additional 25 minutes.
6. Continue turning them over to cook uniformly.
7. Serve with mint chutney or ketchup.

371. Carp fritters

INGREDIENTS

- 10- carp filets
- 3- onions chopped
- 5- green chilies
- 1 ½- tbsp. ginger paste
- 1 ½- tsp. garlic paste
- 1 ½- tsp. salt
- 3- tsp. lemon juice
- 2 tsp. garam masala
- 3- eggs
- 2 ½- tbsp. white sesame seeds

INSTRUCTIONS

1. Blend the ingredients in a bowl.
2. Form this blend into round, flat galettes.
3. Wet the galettes with a small amount of water. Coat each galette with crushed peanuts.
4. Preheat the Air Fryer to 160 F for 5 minutes.
5. Place the galettes in the fry bin and let them cook for an additional 25 minutes.
6. Continue turning them over to cook uniformly.
7. Serve with mint chutney or ketchup.

372. Caribou fingers

INGREDIENTS

- 1 lb. boneless caribou
- 2 cup dry breadcrumbs
- 2 tsp. oregano
- 2 tsp. red chili flakes

Marinade:

- 1 ½- tbsp. ginger-garlic paste
- 4- tbsp. lemon juice
- 2 tsp. salt
- 1 tsp. pepper powder
- 1 tsp. red chili powder
- 6- tbsp. corn flour
- 4- eggs

INSTRUCTIONS

1. Blend all marinade ingredients and soak the meat for 20-30 minutes.
2. Blend the breadcrumbs, oregano and red chili well and dip the marinated fingers in this mix.
3. Preheat the Air Fryer to 160 F for 5 minutes.
4. Cook for 15 minutes, shaking halfway through.

373. Ham Club Sandwich

INGREDIENTS

- 2 slices of white bread
- 1 tbsp. softened butter
- 1 lb. ham
- 1 small capsicum

For Barbeque Sauce:

- ¼- tbsp. Worcestershire sauce
- ½- tsp. olive oil
- ½- flake garlic crushed
- ¼- tsp. mustard powder
- ¼- cup chopped onion
- ½- tbsp. sugar
- 1 tbsp. tomato ketchup
- ¼- tbsp. red chili sauce
- ½- cup water.
- A pinch of salt and black pepper

INSTRUCTIONS

1. Cut the bread diagonally.
2. Cook the sauce ingredients and until it thickens.
3. Add the oyster to the sauce and mix.
4. Cook the capsicum and strip the skin off.
5. Cut the capsicum into strips. Assemble sandwich filling between bread slices.
6. Preheat the air fryer for 5 minutes at 300 F and cook for 15 minutes.
7. Serve the sandwiches with tomato ketchup or mint chutney.

374. Pheasant Chili

INGREDIENTS

- 1 lb. cubed pheasant
- 2 ½- tsp. ginger-garlic paste
- 1 tsp. red chili sauce
- ¼- tsp. salt
- ¼- tsp. red chili powder/black pepper
- Edible orange food coloring

For sauce:

- 2 tbsp. olive oil
- 1 ½- tsp. ginger garlic paste
- ½- tbsp. red chili sauce
- 2 tbsp. tomato ketchup
- 2 tsp. soy sauce
- 1-2- tbsp. honey
- ¼- tsp. Ajinomoto
- 1-2- tsp. red chili flakes

INSTRUCTIONS

1. Blend all of the components for the marinade and marinate veal fingers for 30 minutes.

2. Blend the breadcrumbs, oregano and red chili flakes and add the marinated fingers on this mix.
3. Preheat the Air Fryer to 160 F and cook for 15 minutes, shaking the fry basket occasionally.

375. Duck Liver fries

INGREDIENTS

- 1 lb. duck liver

For the marinade:

- 1 tbsp. olive oil
- 1 tsp. mixed herbs
- ½- tsp. red chili flakes
- A pinch of salt to taste
- 1 tbsp. lemon juice

For the garnish:

- 1 cup melted cheddar

INSTRUCTIONS

1. Blend all marinade ingredients and soak the meat for 20-30 minutes.
2. Blend the breadcrumbs, oregano and red chili well and dip the marinated fingers in this mix.
3. Preheat the Air Fryer to 160 F for 5 minutes. Cook for 15 minutes, shaking halfway through.

376. Ham Pancakes

INGREDIENTS

- 2 tbsp. garam masala
- 1 lb. thinly sliced ham
- 3 tsp ginger finely chopped
- 1-2 tbsp. fresh coriander leaves
- 2 or 3 green chilies
- 1 ½ tbsp. lemon juice
- Salt and pepper to taste

INSTRUCTIONS

1. Blend the ingredients in a bowl and add water to it.
2. Ensure that the paste isn't excessively watery yet is sufficient to apply on the sides of the ham cuts. preheat the Air Fryer to 160 F for 5 minutes.

3. Place the galettes in the fry crate and give them a chance to cook for an additional 25 minutes at a similar temperature.
4. Continue turning them over to cook uniformly.
5. Serve either with mint chutney or ketchup.

377. Clam galette

INGREDIENTS

- 2 tbsp. garam masala
- 1 lb. minced clams
- 3 tsp ginger finely chopped
- 1-2 tbsp. fresh coriander leaves
- 2 or 3 green chilies
- 1 ½ tbsp. lemon juice
- Salt and pepper to taste

INSTRUCTIONS

1. Blend the ingredients in a bowl.
2. Form this blend into round, flat galettes.
3. Wet the galettes with a small amount of water. Coat each galette with crushed peanuts.
4. Preheat the Air Fryer to 160 F for 5 minutes.
5. Place the galettes in the fry bin and let them cook for an additional 25 minutes.
6. Continue turning them over to cook uniformly.
7. Serve with mint chutney or ketchup

378. Pheasant Tikka

INGREDIENTS

- 2 cups sliced pheasant
- 1 large capsicum
- 1 onion
- 5 tbsp. gram flour
- A pinch of salt to taste

For the filling:

- 2 cup fresh green coriander
- ½ cup mint leaves
- 4 tsp. fennel
- 2 tbsp. ginger-garlic paste
- 1 small onion
- 6-7 flakes garlic (optional)
- Salt to taste
- 3 tbsp. lemon juice

INSTRUCTIONS

1. You will start with want to make the chutney.
2. Add the ingredients to a blender and make a thick paste.
3. Cut the bits of fowl and stuff a large portion of the paste into the depression were given.
4. Take the rest of the paste and add it to the gram flour and salt.
5. Toss the bits of chicken on this combination and put it in a safe place.
6. Apply a smidgen of the mixture on the capsicum and onion.
7. Place these on a stick along with the chook pieces.
8. Preheat the Air Fryer to 290 F for around 5 minutes.
9. Open the bin. Organize the satay sticks as they should be.
10. Close the crate. Keep the sticks with the lamb at 180 stages for around half-hour at the same time as the sticks with the vegetables are to be kept at a comparable temperature for simply 7 minutes.
11. Turn the sticks inside the middle of with the intention that one side doesn't get singed and furthermore to offer a uniform cooking.

379.   Seafood Wontons

INGREDIENTS

For dough:

- 1 ½ cup all-purpose flour
- ½ tsp. salt
- 5 tbsp. water
- For filling:
- 2 cups minced seafood
- 2 tbsp. oil
- 2 tsp. ginger-garlic paste
- 2 tsp. soy sauce
- 2 tsp. vinegar

INSTRUCTIONS

1. Mix the dough, cover it with saran wrap and set aside.
2. Mix the filling ingredients.
3. Fold the dough and cut it into a square.
4. Place the filling in the middle.

5. Wrap the dough to cover the filling and squeeze the edges together.
6. Preheat the Air Fryer to 200° F for 5 minutes. Place in the fry bin and cook for 20 minutes.

380.   Squab Cutlet

INGREDIENTS

- 2 lb. boneless squab

1st Marinade:

- 3 tbsp. vinegar or lemon juice
- 2 or 3 tsp. paprika
- 1 tsp. black pepper
- 1 tsp. salt
- 3 tsp. ginger-garlic paste

2nd Marinade:

- 1 cup yogurt
- 4 tsp. tandoori masala
- 2 tbsp. dry fenugreek leaves
- 1 tsp. black salt
- 1 tsp. chat masala
- 1 tsp. garam masala powder
- 1 tsp. red chili powder
- 1 tsp. salt
- 3 drops of red color

INSTRUCTIONS

1. Combine the ingredients. Form round cutlets with the mixture.
2. Preheat the Air Fryer to 250 F for 5 minutes and cook for 10-12 minutes.
3. Serve hot with mint chutney.

381.   Lobster Kebab

INGREDIENTS

- 1 lb. lobster
- 3 onions chopped
- 5 green chilies-roughly chopped
- 1 ½ tbsp. ginger paste
- 1 ½ tsp garlic paste
- 1 ½ tsp salt
- 3 tsp lemon juice
- 2 tsp garam masala
- 4 tbsp. chopped coriander

- 3 tbsp. cream
- 2 tbsp. coriander powder
- 4 tbsp. fresh mint chopped
- 3 tbsp. chopped capsicum
- 3 eggs
- 2 ½ tbsp. white sesame seeds

INSTRUCTIONS

1. Mix the lobster with the ground ginger and cut green chilies.
2. Pound this blend until it turns into a thick paste.
3. Add water if required. Add the onions, mint, breadcrumbs and spices.
4. Blend this well until you get a soft mixture.
5. Form round kebabs with the cough.
6. Pour a small amount of milk onto each kebab to wet it.
7. Roll the kebab in the dry breadcrumbs.
8. Preheat the Air Fryer for 5 minutes at 300 F and cook for 30 minutes.
9. Recommended sides for this dish are mint chutney, tomato ketchup or yogurt chutney.

382. Squab fingers

INGREDIENTS

- ½ lb. squab fingers
- 2 cups of dry breadcrumbs
- 1 cup oil

Marinade:

- 1 ½ tbsp. ginger-garlic paste
- 3 tbsp. lemon juice
- 2 tsp salt
- 1 ½ tsp pepper powder
- 1 tsp red chili flakes
- 3 eggs
- 5 tbsp. corn flour
- 2 tsp tomato ketchup

INSTRUCTIONS

1. Blend all marinade ingredients and soak the meat for 20-30 minutes.
2. Blend the breadcrumbs, oregano and red chili well and dip the marinated fingers in this mix.
3. Preheat the Air Fryer to 160 F for 5 minutes.
4. Cook for 15 minutes, shaking halfway through.

383. Mini Cherry Pies

Total time: 15 minutes

Servings: 6

INGREDIENTS

- 14 0z. Pie crust, refrigerated and thawed
- 1/2 cup pie filling
- 3 tbsp confectioners' sugar
- 1/2 tsp milk
- Cooking spray

INSTRUCTIONS

1. Cut out 6 pies with cookie cutter.
2. Place 1 1/2 tbsp pie filling at the center of each pie pieces.
3. Fold pie in half and seal the seams my pressing with a fork. Make 3 light cuts on top of the pie.
4. Place in air fryer basket and spray with cooking spray.
5. Cook at 175°C for 10 minutes or until lightly brown.
6. Remove and set aside to cool.
7. Mix milk and sugar thoroughly in a small bowl and drizzle over the top of the pies.
8. Serve and enjoy.

384. Air Fryer Cheesecake Bites

Total time: 1 hour

Servings: 4

INGREDIENTS

- 8 oz. cream cheese
- 4 tbsp heavy cream, divided
- 1/2 tsp vanilla extract
- 1/2 cup almond flour
- 1/2 cup erythritol

INSTRUCTIONS

1. Allow cream cheese to sit for 20 minutes at room temperature.
2. Mix cream cheese, erythritol, vanilla concentrate, and 2 tbsp heavy cream in a blender for 3 to 5 minutes or until smooth.
3. Scoop blend into a preparing skillet that has been fixed with a material paper.

4. Freeze blend for 30 minutes or until it structures.
5. Mix almond flour and 2 tbsp erythritol in a little bowl.
6. Dip solidified cheesecake adjusts into staying overwhelming cream and coat in the almond flour blend.
7. Air fry for 2 minutes and serve.

385. Coconut French Toast

Total time: 4 minutes

Servings: 1

INGREDIENTS

- 2 slices gluten free bread
- 1/2 cup shredded coconut
- 1 tbsp baking powder
- 1/2 cup coconut milk
- Maple syrup

INSTRUCTIONS

1. In a large bowl, mix coconut milk and baking powder.
2. Spread shredded coconut on a level sheet.
3. Using every one of the breads, absorb coconut milk before covering in shredded coconut. Coat liberally.
4. Place covered bread in the air fryer bin and air fry at 175°C for 4 minutes.
5. Top with maple syrup.

386. Air Fryer Honey Cheese Balls

Total time: 20 minutes

Servings: 12

INGREDIENTS

- 4 oz. soft goat cheese
- 1 small egg, beaten
- 1 tbsp all-purpose flour
- 1/4 cup breadcrumbs
- 4 tbsp raw honey

INSTRUCTIONS

1. Separate goat cheese into 12 portions and roll into small balls.

2. Freeze balls for about 15 to 20 minutes.
3. Remove from refrigerator and dredge each goat cheese in flour, egg and finally coat then in breadcrumbs.
4. Arrange in air fryer basket and spray with nonstick cooking spray for crispness.
5. Air fry at 200°C for 8 minutes unti golden brown.
6. Drizzle with generous amount of honey and serve immediately.

387. Air Fryer Brownie Bombs
Total time: 40 minutes
Servings: 6

INGREDIENTS

- 1/2 cup chocolate chips
- 4 small eggs
- 1/2 cup Brown sugar
- 1/2 cup butter, unsalted
- 1 tsp vanilla extract
- Olive oil

INSTRUCTIONS

1. Combine butter and chocolate contributes a microwave-safe bowl and microwave for 1 moment and mix.
2. In another bowl, include eggs, sugar and vanilla concentrate and whisk until the blend is sufficiently light.
3. Still whisking, pour in chocolate butter blend and mix well.
4. Grease a 7-inch heating dish with oil.
5. Pour batter into the dish and place container in air fryer.
6. Air fry at 175°C for 25 minutes.

388. Soft Chocolate Cookies
Total time: 15 minutes
Servings: 9

INGREDIENTS

- 100g butter
- 85g brown sugar
- 170g Self Raising Flour
- 100g dark chocolate chips
- 1 tbsp whole milk

INSTRUCTIONS

1. Preheat air fryer to 180°C.
2. In a large bowl, combine butter and sugar, and beat them together until light and fleecy.
3. Stir in flour and blend all together.
4. Crumble the chocolate chips to get a blend of medium and tiny pieces.
5. Add in crushed chocolate and mix.
6. Spoon treats onto a baking sheet and place in air fryer. Cook at 180°C for 6 minutes.
7. After 6 minutes, lower temperature to 160°C for an additional 2 minutes. Serve and enjoy it!

389. Strawberry Almond Bites
Total time: 15 minutes
Servings: 15

INGREDIENTS

- 1 cup oatmeal
- 1/2 cup peanut butter
- 1/3 cup chopped almonds
- 1/3 cup sweetened coconut, shredded
- 1/4 cup honey
- 1/3 cup dried strawberries, chopped

INSTRUCTIONS

1. In an air fryer, heat cereal. almonds and coconut at 175°C for 10 minutes, blending soon after 5 minutes. Enable the blend to cool.
2. In a microwave-safe bowl, microwave the nutty spread for 30 seconds or unt l runny.
3. Add in the prepared blend, honey, and cranberries to the bowl.
4. Form batter into a 1.5-inch balls and refrigerate.

390. Chocolate Mug Cake
Total time: 15 minutes
Servings: 3-4

INGREDIENTS

- 1/4 Cup Self Raising Flour
- 5 tbsp brown sugar
- 1 tbsp Cocoa Powder
- 3 tbsp Milk
- 3 tbsp olive oil

INSTRUCTIONS

1. Mix flour, milk, cocoa powder, sugar and oil together in a mug.
2. Place in the Air fryer and cook at 200°C for about 10 minutes.

391.   Apple Dumplings

Total time: 1 hour
Servings: 1

INGREDIENTS

- 1 small apple, peeled and core removed
- 1 sheet puff pastry
- 1/2 tbsp raisins
- 1/2 tbsp brown sugar
- 1 tbsp melted butter

INSTRUCTIONS

1. Preheat your air fryer to 175°C.
2. Combine raisins and brown sugar in a bowl.
3. Place apple on puff baked accurate sheet and fill the middle with the raisin combo.
4. Crease baked correct over the apple so it's miles very plenty secured.
5. Place dumplings on a baking sheet lined with foil. Brush with melted butter.
6. Place dumplings in air fryer crate and cook for 25 minutes, flipping halfway through.
7. Allow it to cool for 10 minutes before serving.

392.   Molten Lava Cake

Total time: 20 minutes
Servings: 4

INGREDIENTS

- 1 1/2 tbsp self-rising Flour
- 3 tbsp Sugar
- 3 1/2 oz. butter
- 3 oz dark Chocolate
- 2 eggs, beaten

INSTRUCTIONS

1. Preheat Air Fryer To 190°C.
2. Grease and sprinkle, 4 ramekins with flour.
3. In a microwave-safe bowl, dissolve chocolate and butter for around 3 minutes, mixing well.
4. Whisk sugar with eggs until foamy.

5. Pour dissolved chocolate blend into egg blend. Add flour.
6. Pour cake blend into ramekins, around 3/4 full and cook in the preheated air fryer for 10 minutes.

393.   Air Fryer Banana

Total time: 20 minutes
Servings:

INGREDIENTS

- 3 tbsp coconut oil
- 8 ripe Bananas, peeled and halved
- 3 egg whites
- 1/2 cup Corn Flour
- 3 tbsp Cinnamon Sugar
- 1 cup breadcrumbs

INSTRUCTIONS

1. Heat oil in a skillet and add breadcrumbs. Cook for 3-4 minutes.
2. Remove from heat and place in a bowl.
3. Roll every banana half first in corn flour, then in eggs, and lastly in breadcrumbs.
4. Sprinkle with Cinnamon Sugar.
5. Bake at 140°C for 10 minutes.

394.   Pecan Pie

Total time: 25 minutes
Servings: 8

INGREDIENTS

- 1 sheet thawed puff pastry
- 4 tbsp Brown Sugar
- 1/2 butter, melted
- 2 tbsp maple syrup
- 1/2 cup Pecans, chopped

INSTRUCTIONS

1. Combine butter, maple syrup, and chopped pecans in a bowl and place in the freezer for 10 minutes.
2. Unfold puff pastry onto a floured tabletop and cut into equal-sized rectangles.
3. Spoon 2 tsp of filling into one side of each pastry, take the other edge and fold it over pastry.
4. Seal with a fork and pierce each pie.

5. Cook in preheated air fryer 190° C for 7 minutes until golden brown and puffed.

395. Lime Cupcakes

Total time: 32 minutes

Servings: 6

INGREDIENTS:

- 200g soft cheese
- 1/4 cup caster sugar
- 240g Greek yoghurt
- 2 Large Eggs, 1 egg yolk
- 2 limes, juiced

INSTRUCTIONS

1. Mix Greek yogurt and soft cheese together until well blended.
2. Add in eggs and mix again. Then add limes and mix.
3. Fill up 6 cupcake tins with mixture.
4. Bake cupcakes in Air fryer at 160°C for 10 minutes and at 180°C for another 10 minutes.
5. Remove cupcakes from air fryer and allow to cool for 8 to 10 minutes
6. Refrigerate for 4 hours. Top with remaining limes and serve.

396. Banana Croquette

INGREDIENTS

- 2 cups sliced banana
- 3 onions chopped
- 5 green chilies-roughly chopped
- 1 ½ tbsp. ginger paste
- 1 ½ tsp. garlic paste
- 1 ½ tsp. salt
- 3 tsp. lemon juice
- 2 tsp. garam masala
- 4 tbsp. chopped coriander
- 3 tbsp. cream
- 3 tbsp. chopped capsicum
- 3 eggs
- 2 ½ tbsp. white sesame seeds

INSTRUCTIONS

1. Crush the ingredients aside from the banana and egg and create a smooth paste.

2. Coat the banana in the paste. Presently, beat the eggs and add somewhat salt to it.
3. Beat the eggs and add salt.
4. Dip the bananas in the egg blend and then coat with sesame seeds. Place on skewers.
5. Preheat the Air Fryer to 160 F and cook for 25 minutes.
6. Turn the sticks over in the middle of the cooking procedure to cook uniformly.

397. Apricot Kebab

INGREDIENTS

- 2 cups fresh apricots
- 3 onions chopped
- 5 green chilies-roughly chopped
- 1 ½ tbsp. ginger paste
- 1 ½ tsp. garlic paste
- 1 ½ tsp. salt
- 3 tsp. lemon juice
- 2 tsp. garam masala
- 3 eggs
- 2 ½ tbsp. white sesame seeds

INSTRUCTIONS

1. Crush the ingredients aside from the apricot and egg and make a smooth paste.
2. Coat the apricots in the paste. Beat the eggs and add salt.
3. Dip the apricots in the egg blend and then coat with sesame seeds.
4. Place on skewers.
5. Preheat the Air Fryer to 160 F and cook for 25 minutes.
6. Turn the sticks over in the middle of the cooking procedure to cook uniform y.

398. Strawberry Tarts

INGREDIENTS

- 1 ½ cup plain flour
- 3 tbsp. unsalted butter
- 2 tbsp. powdered sugar
- 2 cups cold water

Filling:

- 2 cups sliced strawberries
- 1 cup fresh cream

- 3 tbsp. butter

INSTRUCTIONS

1. In a large bowl, blend the flour, cocoa powder, butter and sugar.
2. Press crust into the baking tin and leave it to cool for ten minutes.
3. Mix the filling ingredients in a bowl. Ensure that it is somewhat thick.
4. Preheat the fryer to 300 F. Cook for 15 minutes or until golden brown.
5. Slice and serve with whipped cream.

399. Strawberry Pudding

INGREDIENTS

- 1 cup strawberry juice
- 2 cups milk
- 2 tbsp. custard powder
- 3 tbsp. powdered sugar
- 3 tbsp. unsalted butter
- 1 cup strawberry slices

INSTRUCTIONS

1. Heat the milk and sugar and add the custard powder, then strawberry juice and mix till you get a thick blend.
2. Preheat the air fryer to 300 F for 5 minutes.
3. Place the dish in the container and lower the temperature to 250 F.
4. Cook for ten minutes and set aside to cool.
5. Garnish with strawberries.

400. Banana Pudding

INGREDIENTS

- 1 cup banana juice
- 2 cups milk
- 2 tbsp. custard powder
- 3 tbsp. powdered sugar
- 3 tbsp. unsalted butter
- 3 tbsp. chopped mixed nuts

INSTRUCTIONS

1. Heat the milk and sugar and add the custard powder, then banana juice and mix till you get a thick blend.

2. Preheat the air fryer to 300 F for 5 minutes.
3. Place the dish in the container and lower the temperature to 250 F.
4. Cook for ten minutes and set aside to cool.
5. Garnish with nuts.

401. Almond Milk Pudding

INGREDIENTS

- 2 cups almond powder
- 2 cups milk
- 1 tsp. gelatin
- 2 tbsp. custard powder
- 3 tbsp. powdered sugar
- 3 tbsp. unsalted butter

INSTRUCTIONS

1. Heat the milk and sugar and add the custard powder, then almond powder and gelatin and mix till you get a thick blend.
2. Preheat the air fryer to 300 F for 5 minutes.
3. Place the dish in the container and lower the temperature to 250 F.
4. Cook for ten minutes and set aside to cool.

402. Bebinca

INGREDIENTS

- 1 cup coconut milk
- 1 cup almond flour
- 2 cups milk
- 2 tbsp. custard powder
- 3 tbsp. powdered sugar
- 3 tbsp. unsalted butter

INSTRUCTIONS

1. Heat the milk and sugar and add the custard powder, then flour and mix till you get a thick blend.
2. Preheat the air fryer to 300 F for 5 minutes. Place the dish in the container and lower the temperature to 250 F. Cook for ten minutes and set aside to cool. Garnish with strawberries.

403. Creamy caramel pudding

INGREDIENTS

- 2 cups milk
- 2 cups custard powder
- 3 tbsp. powdered sugar
- 3 tbsp. unsalted butter
- 4 tbsp. caramel

INSTRUCTIONS

1. Heat the milk and sugar and add the custard powder, then almond powder and gelatin and mix till you get a thick blend.
2. Preheat the air fryer to 300 F for 5 minutes.
3. Place the dish in the container and lower the temperature to 250 F.
4. Cook for ten minutes and set aside to cool.
5. Spread caramel over the dish and serve warm.

404. Honey and Orange Pancakes

INGREDIENTS

- 1 orange (zested)
- 1 ½ cups almond flour
- 3 eggs
- 1 tbsp. honey
- 2 tsp. dried basil
- 2 tsp. dried parsley
- Salt and Pepper to taste
- 3 tbsp. Butter

INSTRUCTIONS

1. Preheat the air fryer to 250 F.
2. In a small bowl, combine the ingredients. Mix well.
3. Cook till both sides of the pancake have browned. Serve with maple syrup.

405. Fig Pudding

INGREDIENTS

- 2 cups milk
- 2 cups almond flour
- 2 tbsp. custard powder
- 3 tbsp. powdered sugar
- 3 tbsp. unsalted butter
- 2 cups figs

INSTRUCTIONS

1. Heat the milk and sugar and add the custard powder, then almond flower and mix till you get a thick blend.
2. Preheat the air fryer to 300 F for 5 minutes.
3. Place the dish in the container and lower the temperature to 250 F.
4. Cook for ten minutes and set aside to cool.

406. Apricot Pudding

INGREDIENTS

- 2 cups almond flour
- 2 cups milk
- 2 tbsp. custard powder
- 3 tbsp. powdered sugar
- 3 tbsp. unsalted butter
- 2 cups apricot

INSTRUCTIONS

1. Heat the milk and sugar and add the custard powder, then almond flower and apricot and mix till you get a thick blend.
2. Preheat the air fryer to 300 F for 5 minutes.
3. Place the dish in the container and lower the temperature to 250 F.
4. Cook for ten minutes and set aside to cool.

407. Baked Cream

INGREDIENTS

For the cream:

- 2 cups condensed milk
- 2 cups fresh cream
- For garnishing:
- 1 cup fresh strawberries
- 1 cup fresh blueberries
- 1 cup blackberries
- Handful of mint leaves
- 3 tsp. sugar
- 4 tsp. water

INSTRUCTIONS

1. Blend the cream and add the milk to it.

2. Whisk the ingredients well together and move this mix into small warming dishes promising you don't overburden the dishes.
3. Preheat the fryer to 300 F for 5 minutes.
4. You should place the dishes in the container and spread it.
5. Cook it for 15 minutes. Exactly when you shake the dishes, the mix ought to just shake yet not break.
6. Leave it in the ice chest to set and subsequently coordinate the normal items, ingredients and serve.

408. Pistachio Pudding

INGREDIENTS

- 2 cups milk
- 2 cups almond flour
- 2 tbsp. custard powder
- 3 tbsp. powdered sugar
- 3 tbsp. unsalted butter
- 2 cups finely chopped pistachio

INSTRUCTIONS

1. Heat the milk and sugar and add the custard powder, then almond flower and pistachio and mix till you get a thick blend.
2. Preheat the air fryer to 300 F for 5 minutes.
3. Place the dish in the container and lower the temperature to 250 F.
4. Cook for ten minutes and set aside to cool.

409. Orange & Persimmon Pudding

INGREDIENTS

- 2 cups milk
- 2 cups almond flour
- 2 tbsp. custard powder
- 3 tbsp. powdered sugar
- 3 tbsp. unsalted butter
- 2 oranges (sliced)
- 2 persimmons (sliced)

INSTRUCTIONS

1. Heat the milk and sugar and add the custard powder, then almond powder and fruit and mix till you get a thick blend.
2. Preheat the air fryer to 300 F for 5 minutes.

3. Place the dish in the container and lower the temperature to 250 F.
4. Cook for ten minutes and set aside to cool.

410. Blueberry Pudding

INGREDIENTS

- 1 cup blueberry juice
- 2 cups milk
- 2 tbsp. custard powder
- 3 tbsp. powdered sugar
- 3 tbsp. unsalted butter

INSTRUCTIONS

1. Heat the milk and sugar and add the custard powder, then blueberry juice and mix till you get a thick blend.
2. Preheat the air fryer to 300 F for 5 minutes.
3. Place the dish in the container and lower the temperature to 250 F.
4. Cook for ten minutes and set aside to cool.

411. Po'e

INGREDIENTS

- 2 cups coconut milk
- 1 cup fresh cream
- 2 tbsp. custard powder
- 3 tbsp. powdered sugar
- 3 tbsp. unsalted butter
- 1 cup pineapple slices
- 1 cup mango slices
- 1 cup banana slices

INSTRUCTIONS

1. Heat the milk and sugar and add the custard powder, then fresh cream and fruit and mix till you get a thick blend.
2. Preheat the air fryer to 300 F for 5 minutes.
3. Place the dish in the container and lower the temperature to 250 F.
4. Cook for ten minutes and set aside to cool.

412. Mini Pancakes

INGREDIENTS

- 1 ½ cups almond flour

- 3 eggs
- 2 tsp. dried basil
- 2 tsp. dried parsley
- Salt and Pepper to taste
- 3 tbsp. Butter

INSTRUCTIONS

1. Preheat the air fryer to 250 F.
2. In a small bowl, combine the ingredients. Mix well.
3. Cook till both sides of the pancake have browned. Serve with maple syrup.

413. Rice pudding

INGREDIENTS

- 2 cups milk
- 2 tbsp. custard powder
- 3 tbsp. powdered sugar
- 2 tbsp. rice
- 3 tbsp. unsalted butter

INSTRUCTIONS

1. Heat the milk and sugar and add the custard powder, then rice and mix til you get a thick blend.
2. Preheat the air fryer to 300 F for 5 minutes.
3. Place the dish in the container and lower the temperature to 250 F.
4. Cook for ten minutes and set aside to cool.

414. Sago Payasam

INGREDIENTS

- 2 cups milk
- 2 cups-soaked sago
- 2 tbsp. custard powder
- 3 tbsp. powdered sugar
- 3 tbsp. unsalted butter

INSTRUCTIONS

1. Heat the milk and sugar and add the custard powder, then sago and mix til you get a thick blend.
2. Preheat the air fryer to 300 F for 5 minutes.
3. Place the dish in the container and lower the temperature to 250 F.

4. Cook for ten minutes and set aside to cool.

415. Cardamom Cupcakes

INGREDIENTS

- 2 cups All-purpose flour
- 1 ½ cup milk
- 1 tbsp. cardamom powder
- ½ tsp. baking powder
- ½ tsp. baking soda
- 2 tbsp. butter
- 2 tbsp. sugar
- Muffin cups

INSTRUCTIONS

1. Combine the ingredients except milk to create a crumbly blend.
2. Add this milk to the blend and make a batter and pour into the muffin cups.
3. Preheat the fryer to 300 F and cook 15 minutes.
4. Check whether they are done using a toothpick.

416. Cranberry Pancakes

INGREDIENTS

- 2 cups minced cranberry
- 1 ½ cups almond flour
- 3 eggs
- 2 tsp. dried basil
- 2 tsp. dried parsley
- Salt and Pepper to taste
- 3 tbsp. Butter

INSTRUCTIONS

1. Preheat the air fryer to 250 F.
2. In a small bowl, combine the ingredients. Mix well.
3. Cook till both sides of the pancake have browned.
4. Serve with maple syrup.

417. Vanilla Pudding

INGREDIENTS

- 2 cups milk

- 2 cups almond flour
- 1 tbsp. vanilla essence
- 2 tbsp. custard powder
- 3 tbsp. powdered sugar
- 3 tbsp. unsalted butter

INSTRUCTIONS

1. Heat the milk and sugar and add the custard powder, then almond flour and vanilla and mix till you get a thick blend.
2. Preheat the air fryer to 300 F for 5 minutes.
3. Place the dish in the container and lower the temperature to 250 F.
4. Cook for ten minutes and set aside to cool.

418. Chocolate Chip Waffles

INGREDIENTS

- 3 cups cocoa powder
- 3 eggs
- 2 tsp. dried basil
- 2 tsp. dried parsley
- Salt and Pepper to taste
- 3 tbsp. Butter
- 1 cup chocolate chips

INSTRUCTIONS

1. Preheat the air fryer to 250 F.
2. In a small bowl, mix the ingredients, except the chocolate chips.
3. Take a waffle shape and grease it with butter.
4. Pour the batter and cook till both sides have browned.
5. Top with chocolate chips and serve.

419. Saffron Pudding

INGREDIENTS

- 2 cups milk
- 2 tbsp. saffron
- 2 cups almond flour
- 2 tbsp. custard powder
- 3 tbsp. powdered sugar
- 3 tbsp. unsalted butter

INSTRUCTIONS

1. Heat the milk and sugar and add the custard powder, then almond flour and saffron and mix till you get a thick blend.
2. Preheat the air fryer to 300 F for 5 minutes.
3. Place the dish in the container and lower the temperature to 250 F.
4. Cook for ten minutes and set aside to cool.

420. Zucchini Pancakes

INGREDIENTS

- 2 zucchinis
- 1 ½ cups almond flour
- 3 eggs
- 2 tsp. dried basil
- 2 tsp. dried parsley
- Salt and Pepper to taste
- 3 tbsp. Butter

INSTRUCTIONS

1. Preheat the air fryer to 250 F.
2. In a small bowl, combine the ingredients. Mix well.
3. Cook till both sides of the pancake have browned.
4. Serve with maple syrup.

421. Upside Down Pineapple Cake

INGREDIENTS

For the batter:

- 2 tbsp. butter
- ¼ cup condensed milk
- 2 tsp. pineapple essence
- 2 cups All Purpose Flour
- ¼ tsp. baking powder
- ¼ tsp. baking soda
- ½ cup drinking soda
- ½ tbsp. powdered sugar
- 3 tbsp. sugar
- 8 cherries

INSTRUCTIONS

1. Grease the tin with butter and line it with wax paper.
2. Dust the tin with the flour.

3. Add the slices of the pineapple to the base of the tin.
4. Melt the sugar and make it into the caramel. Pour this caramel into the tin.
5. Mix the batter ingredients in a large bowl. Beat till you get a uniform batter.
6. Pour the batter into the tin.
7. Preheat the fryer to 300 F and cook the cake for 15 minutes.
8. Check whether the cake is done using a toothpick.

422. Chocolate Tarts

INGREDIENTS

- 1 ½ cup plain flour
- ½ cup cocoa powder
- 3 tbsp. unsalted butter
- 2 tbsp. powdered sugar
- 2 cups cold water
- 1 tbsp. sliced cashew
- For Truffle filling:
- 1 ½ melted chocolate
- 1 cup fresh cream
- 3 tbsp. butter

INSTRUCTIONS

1. In a large bowl, blend the flour, cocoa powder, butter and sugar.
2. Press crust into the baking tin and leave it to cool for ten minutes.
3. Mix the filling ingredients in a bowl. Ensure that it is somewhat thick.
4. Preheat the fryer to 300 F. Cook for 15 minutes or until golden brown.
5. Slice and serve with whipped cream.

423. Vanilla and Oat Pudding

INGREDIENTS

- 2 cups vanilla powder
- 2 cups milk
- 1 cup oats
- 2 tbsp. custard powder
- 3 tbsp. powdered sugar
- 3 tbsp. unsalted butter

INSTRUCTIONS

1. Heat the milk and sugar and add the custard powder, then oats and vanilla powder and mix till you get a thick blend.
2. Preheat the air fryer to 300 F for 5 minutes.
3. Place the dish in the container and lower the temperature to 250 F.
4. Cook for ten minutes and set aside to cool.

424. Blueberry Cupcakes

INGREDIENTS

- 2 cups All-purpose flour
- 1 ½ cup milk
- ½ tsp. baking powder
- ½ tsp. baking soda
- 2 tbsp. butter
- 1 cup sugar
- 3 tsp. vinegar
- 2 cups blueberries
- ½ tsp. vanilla essence
- Muffin cups or butter paper cups.

INSTRUCTIONS

1. Combine the ingredients except milk to create a crumbly blend.
2. Add this milk to the blend and make a batter and pour into the muffin cups.
3. Preheat the fryer to 300 F and cook 15 minutes.
4. Check whether they are done using a toothpick.

425. Chocolate Chip Muffins

INGREDIENTS

- 2 cups All-purpose flour
- 1 ½ cup milk
- ½ tsp. baking powder
- ½ tsp. baking soda
- 2 tbsp. butter
- 1 cup sugar
- 3 tsp. vinegar
- ½ cup chocolate chips
- ½ tsp. vanilla essence
- Muffin cups or butter paper cups

INSTRUCTIONS

1. Combine the ingredients except milk to create a crumbly blend.
2. Add this milk to the blend and make a batter and pour into the muffin cups.
3. Preheat the fryer to 300 F and cook 15 minutes.
4. Check whether they are done using a toothpick.

426. Strawberry Pancakes

INGREDIENTS

- 2 cups minced strawberries
- 1 ½ cups almond flour
- 3 eggs
- 2 tsp. dried basil
- 2 tsp. dried parsley
- Salt and Pepper to taste
- 3 tbsp. Butter

INSTRUCTIONS

1. Preheat the air fryer to 250 F.
2. In a small bowl, combine the ingredients. Mix well.
3. Cook till both sides of the pancake have browned.
4. Serve with maple syrup.

427. Orange Muffins

INGREDIENTS

- 2 cups All-purpose flour
- 1 ½ cup milk
- ½ tsp. baking powder
- ½ tsp. baking soda
- 2 tbsp. butter
- 2 tbsp. sugar
- 2 tsp. vinegar
- 3 tbsp. orange juice and zest
- Muffin cups

INSTRUCTIONS

1. Combine the ingredients into a batter.
2. Pour into the muffin cups.
3. Preheat the fryer to 300 F and cook for 15 minutes.
4. Check whether the biscuits are cooked using a toothpick.

428. Cookie Custard

INGREDIENTS

- 1 cup all-purpose flour
- ½ cup icing sugar
- ½ cup custard powder
- 2 tbsp. butter
- A pinch of baking soda and baking powder

INSTRUCTIONS

1. Cream the butter and sugar together. Mix in the rest of the ingredients.
2. Make balls out of the mixture, cover them with flour and place them on a greased baking sheet.
3. Preheat the fryer to 300 F and cook for 20-25 minutes.

429. Chocolate Sponge Cake

INGREDIENTS

- ½ cup condensed milk
- 1 cup all-purpose flour
- ½ cup cocoa powder
- ½ tsp. baking soda
- ½ tsp. baking powder
- ½ cup oil
- 3 tbsp. powdered sugar
- ½ cup soda
- 1 tsp. vanilla essence
- Butter paper to line the tin

INSTRUCTIONS

1. Combine the ingredients to make a batter that is smooth and thick.
2. Oil a cake tin with butter and line it with wax paper.
3. Pour the batter into the tin.
4. Preheat the air fryer to 300 F and cook for 15 minutes.

430. Pumpkin Pancakes

INGREDIENTS

- 1 large pumpkin

- 1 ½ cups almond flour
- 3 eggs
- 2 tsp. dried basil
- 2 tsp. dried parsley
- Salt and Pepper to taste
- 3 tbsp. Butter

INSTRUCTIONS

1. Preheat the air fryer to 250 F.
2. In a small bowl, combine the ingredients. Mix well.
3. Cook till both sides of the pancake have browned. Serve with maple syrup.

431.   Baked Yogurt

INGREDIENTS

For the yoghurt:

- 2 cups condensed milk
- 2 cups yogurt
- 2 cups fresh cream

For garnishing:

- 1 cup fresh strawberries
- 1 cup fresh blueberries
- 1 cup blackberries
- Handful of mint leaves
- 3 tsp. sugar
- 4 tsp. water

INSTRUCTIONS

1. Combine the ingredients and make a thick mix.
2. Preheat the fryer to 300 F and cook for 15 minutes.
3. Refrigerate to set, add garnish and serve.

432.   Nan Khatai

INGREDIENTS

- 1 ½ cup all-purpose flour
- 1 cup Gram flour
- 1 cup +3 tbsp. icing sugar
- 1 tbsp. Unsalted Butter
- 1 tsp. baking powder
- 1 tsp. baking soda

- 1 tsp. cardamom powder

INSTRUCTIONS

1. Mix the ingredients and form small balls.
2. Preheat the fryer to 300 F.
3. Place the prepared baking dish in the bin and lower the temperature to 250 F.
4. Cook for 5 minutes on each side.

433.   Banana Pancakes

INGREDIENTS

- 4 ripe bananas (shredded)
- 1 ½ cups almond flour
- 3 eggs
- 2 tsp. dried basil
- 2 tsp. dried parsley
- Salt and Pepper to taste
- 3 tbsp. Butter

INSTRUCTIONS

1. Preheat the air fryer to 250 F.
2. In a small bowl, combine the ingredients. Mix well.
3. Cook till both sides of the pancake have browned.
4. Serve with maple syrup.

434.   Tapioca Pudding

INGREDIENTS

- 2 cups tapioca pearls
- 2 cups milk
- 2 tbsp. custard powder
- 3 tbsp. powdered sugar
- 3 tbsp. unsalted butter

INSTRUCTIONS

1. Heat the milk and sugar and add the custard powder, then tapioca pearls and mix till you get a thick blend.
2. Preheat the air fryer to 300 F for 5 minutes.
3. Place the dish in the container and lower the temperature to 250 F.
4. Cook for ten minutes and set aside to cool.

435. Oat Muffins

INGREDIENTS

- 2 cups All-purpose flour
- 1 ½ cup milk
- ½ tsp. baking powder
- ½ tsp. baking soda
- 2 tbsp. butter
- 1 cup sugar
- 3 tsp. vinegar
- 1 cup oats
- ½ tsp. vanilla essence
- Butter paper cups.

INSTRUCTIONS

1. Combine the ingredients except milk to create a crumbly blend.
2. Add this milk to the blend and make a batter and pour into the muffin cups.
3. Preheat the fryer to 300 F and cook 15 minutes.
4. Check whether they are done using a toothpick.

436. Honey and Oat Cookie

INGREDIENTS

- 1 cup all-purpose flour
- 1 cups flour
- ½ cup oats
- 1 tsp. baking powder
- 1 tbsp. liquid glucose
- 2 tbsp. powdered sugar
- ½ cup milk
- 1 tbsp. unsalted butter
- 2 tsp. honey

INSTRUCTIONS

1. Combine the dry ingredients in a large bowl and warm the glucose with a little water.
2. Blend the glucose, honey and butter to the bowl with the milk.
3. Roll out the mixture with a rolling pin. Form cookies.
4. Preheat the fryer to 300 F for 5 minutes.
5. Place the prepared baking tin in the container and lower the temperature to 250 F.
6. Cook for 20 minutes.

437. Muffins and Jam

INGREDIENTS

- 2 cup powdered sugar
- 2 cups all-purpose flour
- 1 tsp. baking powder
- ½ tsp. baking soda
- 2 tbsp. jam
- 1 tbsp. unsalted butter
- 2 cups buttermilk
- Parchment paper

INSTRUCTIONS

1. Combine the ingredients except milk to create a crumbly blend.
2. Add this milk to the blend and make a batter and pour into the muffin cups.
3. Preheat the fryer to 300 F and cook 15 minutes.
4. Check whether they are done using a toothpick.
5. Spread jam on top.

438. Fruit Tarts

INGREDIENTS

- 1 ½ cup plain flour
- ½ cup cocoa powder
- 3 tbsp. unsalted butter
- 2 tbsp. powdered sugar
- 2 cups cold water
- 1 tbsp. sliced cashew
- For Truffle filling:
- 2 cups mixed sliced fruits
- 1 cup fresh cream
- 3 tbsp. butter

INSTRUCTIONS

1. In a large bowl, blend the flour, cocoa powder, butter and sugar.
2. Press crust into the baking tin and leave it to cool for ten minutes.
3. Mix the filling ingredients in a bowl. Ensure that it is somewhat thick.
4. Preheat the fryer to 300 F. Cook for 15 minutes or until golden brown.
5. Slice and serve with whipped cream.

439. Bread Pudding

INGREDIENTS

- 6 slices bread
- 2 cups milk
- 2 tbsp. custard powder
- 3 tbsp. powdered sugar
- 3 tbsp. unsalted butter

INSTRUCTIONS

1. Heat the milk and sugar and add the custard powder, then bread slices and mix till you get a thick blend.
2. Preheat the air fryer to 300 F for 5 minutes.
3. Place the dish in the container and lower the temperature to 250 F.
4. Cook for ten minutes and set aside to cool.

440. Chocolate Pudding

INGREDIENTS

- 2 cups of cocoa powder
- 2 cups milk
- 2 tbsp. custard powder
- 3 tbsp. powdered sugar
- 3 tbsp. unsalted butter

INSTRUCTIONS

1. Heat the milk and sugar and add the custard powder, then cocoa powder and mix till you get a thick blend.
2. Preheat the air fryer to 300 F for 5 minutes.
3. Place the dish in the container and lower the temperature to 250 F.
4. Cook for ten minutes and set aside to cool.

441. Cucumber Pancakes

INGREDIENTS

- 5 medium cucumbers (shredded)
- 1 ½ cups almond flour
- 3 eggs
- 2 tsp. dried basil
- 2 tsp. dried parsley
- Salt and Pepper to taste
- 3 tbsp. Butter

INSTRUCTIONS

1. Preheat the air fryer to 250 F.
2. In a small bowl, combine the ingredients. Mix well.
3. Cook till both sides of the pancake have browned.
4. Serve with maple syrup.

442. Vanilla Brownies

INGREDIENTS

- 1 tbsp. unsalted butter
- 2 tbsp. water
- ½ cup chopped nuts
- 3 tbsp. vanilla essence
- 2 cups all-purpose flour
- ½ cup condensed milk

INSTRUCTIONS

1. Include the ingredients together and rush till you get a smooth blend.
2. Set up a tin by lubing it with spread.
3. Move the blend into the tin. Preheat the fryer to 300 F for 5 minutes.
4. You should put the tin in the basket and spread it.
5. Check whether the brownies have been cooked utilizing a blade or a toothpick and remove the plate.
6. At the point when the brownies have cooled, cut them and present with a place of frozen yogurt.

443. Apple Pie

INGREDIENTS

- 1 cup plain flour
- 1 tbsp. unsalted butter
- 4tsp. powdered sugar
- 2 cups cold milk
- For Apple filling:
- ½ cup roasted nuts
- 3 apples
- 2 tbsp. sugar
- ½ tsp. cinnamon
- 2 tsp. lemon juice

INSTRUCTIONS

1. Mix the first four ingredients together to create a dough. Roll the batter out into 2 large circles.
2. Press one circle into the pie tin and prick the sides with a fork.
3. Cook the filling ingredients over low heat and pour it in the tin.
4. Cover the pie tin with the second circle.
5. Preheat the fryer to 300 F for 5 minutes.
6. Cook until golden brown, then let it cool.
7. Slice and serve with a dab of cream.

444. Strawberry Muffins

INGREDIENTS

- 2 cups All-purpose flour
- 1 ½ cup milk
- ½ tsp. baking powder
- ½ tsp. baking soda
- 2 tbsp. butter
- 1 cup sugar
- 3 tsp. vinegar
- ½ cup chocolate chips
- ½ tsp. vanilla essence
- Muffin cups or butter paper cups

INSTRUCTIONS

1. Combine the ingredients except milk to create a crumbly blend.
2. Add this milk to the blend and make a batter and pour into the muffin cups.
3. Preheat the fryer to 300 F and cook 15 minutes.
4. Check whether they are done using a toothpick.

445. Honey and Nut Pie

INGREDIENTS

- 1 cup plain flour
- 1 tbsp. unsalted butter
- 4tsp. powdered sugar
- 2 cups cold milk

For Honey and Nut filling:

- 1 cup roasted mixed nuts
- 3 tbsp. honey
- 2 tbsp. sugar
- ½ tsp. cinnamon
- 2 tsp. lemon juice

INSTRUCTIONS

1. Mix the first four ingredients together to create a dough.
2. Roll the batter out into 2 large circles. Press one circle into the pie tin and prick the sides with a fork.
3. Cook the filling ingredients over low heat and pour it in the tin.
4. Cover the pie tin with the second circle.
5. Preheat the fryer to 300 F for 5 minutes.
6. Cook until golden brown, then let it cool.
7. Slice and serve with a dab of cream.

446. Coconut and Plantain Pancakes

INGREDIENTS

- 2 fresh plantains (shredded)
- 1 cup shredded coconut
- 1 ½ cups almond flour
- 3 eggs
- 2 tsp. dried basil
- 2 tsp. dried parsley
- Salt and Pepper to taste
- 3 tbsp. Butter

INSTRUCTIONS

1. Preheat the air fryer to 250 F.
2. In a small bowl, combine the ingredients. Mix well.
3. Cook till both sides of the pancake have browned. Serve with maple syrup.

447. Vegetable and Oat Muffins

INGREDIENTS

- 2 cup whole wheat flour
- 1 ½ cup milk
- ½ tsp. baking powder
- ½ tsp. baking soda
- 2 tbsp. butter
- 1 cup + 3 tsp. sugar
- 3 tsp. vinegar
- ½ cup oats

- 1 cup mixed vegetables
- ½ tsp. vanilla essence
- Butter paper cups.

INSTRUCTIONS

1. Combine the ingredients except milk to create a crumbly blend.
2. Add this milk to the blend and make a batter and pour into the muffin cups.
3. Preheat the fryer to 300 F and cook 15 minutes.
4. Check whether they are done using a toothpick.

448. **Apricot Blackberry Crumble**

INGREDIENTS

- 2 cups fresh apricots
- 2 cups fresh blackberries
- 1 cup sugar
- 3 tsp. lemon juice
- 1 ½ cups flour
- 3 tbsp. unsalted butter

INSTRUCTIONS

1. Preheat the fryer to 300 F.
2. Cut the fruits and place them in a bowl along with half the sugar and lemon juice.
3. Mix the ingredients well and scoop them into an oven dish and spread them out.
4. In another bowl, mix the flour with remaining sugar, followed by the butter and 2 tbsp. water.
5. Make sure that the mixture is crumbly.
6. Put the dish in the basket and bake for twenty minutes until the rings have turned golden brown.
7. Serve warm.

449. **Bacon and Egg Pie**

INGREDIENTS

- 1 ½ cup plain flour
- 3 tbsp. unsalted butter
- 2 tbsp. powdered sugar
- 2 cups cold water
- 1 tbsp. sliced cashew

Filling:

- 1 cup scrambled egg
- 8 slices bacon
- 3 tbsp. butter

INSTRUCTIONS

1. Mix the first four ingredients together to create a dough.
2. Roll the batter out into 2 large circles.
3. Press one circle into the pie tin and prick the sides with a fork.
4. Cook the filling ingredients over low heat and pour it in the tin.
5. Cover the pie tin with the second circle.
6. Preheat the fryer to 300 F for 5 minutes. Cook until golden brown, then let t cool
7. Slice and serve with a dab of cream.

450. **Banoffee Pie**

INGREDIENTS

- 1 ½ cup plain flour
- 3 tbsp. unsalted butter
- 2 tbsp. powdered sugar
- 2 cups cold water
- 1 tbsp. sliced cashew

Filling:

- 2 cups sliced banana
- 1 cup toffee
- 1 cup fresh cream
- 3 tbsp. butter

INSTRUCTIONS

1. Mix the first four ingredients together to create a dough.
2. Roll the batter out into 2 large circles.
3. Press one circle into the pie tin and prick the sides with a fork.
4. Cook the filling ingredients over low heat and pour it in the tin.
5. Cover the pie tin with the second circle.
6. Preheat the fryer to 300 F for 5 minutes.
7. Cook until golden brown, then let it cool.
8. Slice and serve with a dab of cream.

451. Banana Cream Pie

INGREDIENTS

- 1 ½ cup plain flour
- 3 tbsp. unsalted butter
- 2 tbsp. powdered sugar
- 2 cups cold water
- 1 tbsp. sliced cashew

Filling:

- 2 cups sliced banana
- 1 cup fresh cream
- 3 tbsp. butter

INSTRUCTIONS

1. Mix the first four ingredients together to create a dough.
2. Roll the batter out into 2 large circles.
3. Press one circle into the pie tin and prick the sides with a fork.
4. Cook the filling ingredients over low heat and pour it in the tin.
5. Cover the pie tin with the second circle.
6. Preheat the fryer to 300 F for 5 minutes.
7. Cook until golden brown, then let it cool.
8. Slice and serve with a dab of cream.

452. Kidney Bean Tarts

INGREDIENTS

- 1 ½ cup plain flour
- 3 tbsp. unsalted butter
- 2 tbsp. powdered sugar
- 2 cups cold water
- 1 tbsp. sliced cashew

Filling:

- 2 cups mashed kidney beans
- 1 cup fresh cream
- 3 tbsp. butter

INSTRUCTIONS

1. In a large bowl, blend the flour, cocoa powder, butter and sugar.
2. Press crust into the baking tin and leave it to cool for ten minutes.

3. Mix the filling ingredients in a bowl. Ensure that it is somewhat thick.
4. Preheat the fryer to 300 F. Cook for 15 minutes or until golden brown.
5. Slice and serve with whipped cream.

453. Bisteeya

INGREDIENTS

- 1 ½ cup almond flour
- 3 tbsp. unsalted butter
- 2 tbsp. powdered sugar
- 2 cups cold water
- 1 tbsp. sliced cashew

Filling:

- 2 cups minced chicken
- 1 cup sliced almonds
- 3 tbsp. butter

INSTRUCTIONS

1. Mix the first four ingredients together to create a dough. Roll the batter out into 2 large circles.
2. Press one circle into the pie tin and prick the sides with a fork.
3. Cook the filling ingredients over low heat and pour it in the tin.
4. Cover the pie tin with the second circle.
5. Preheat the fryer to 300 F for 5 minutes.
6. Cook until golden brown, then let it cool.
7. Slice and serve with a dab of cream.

454. Blueberry Tarts

INGREDIENTS

- 1 ½ cup plain flour
- 3 tbsp. unsalted butter
- 2 tbsp. powdered sugar
- 2 cups cold water
- 1 tbsp. sliced cashew

Filling:

- 1 cup fresh blueberries (Sliced)
- 1 cup fresh cream
- 3 tbsp. butter

INSTRUCTIONS

1. In a large bowl, blend the flour, cocoa powder, butter and sugar.
2. Press crust into the baking tin and leave it to cool for ten minutes.
3. Mix the filling ingredients in a bowl. Ensure that it is somewhat thick.
4. Preheat the fryer to 300 F. Cook for 15 minutes or until golden brown.
5. Slice and serve with whipped cream.

455. Bougatsa

INGREDIENTS

- 1 ½ cup plain flour
- 2 tbsp. custard powder
- 3 tbsp. unsalted butter
- 2 tbsp. powdered sugar
- 2 cups cold water
- 1 tbsp. sliced cashew

Filling:

- 2 cups minced meat
- 1 cup Cheddar(melted)
- 1 cup fresh cream
- 3 tbsp. butter

INSTRUCTIONS

1. Mix the first four ingredients together to create a dough.
2. Roll the batter out into 2 large circles.
3. Press one circle into the pie tin and prick the sides with a fork.
4. Cook the filling ingredients over low heat and pour it in the tin.
5. Cover the pie tin with the second circle.
6. Preheat the fryer to 300 F for 5 minutes.
7. Cook until golden brown, then let it cool.
8. Slice and serve with a dab of cream.

456. Buko Pie

INGREDIENTS

- 1 ½ cup plain flour
- 3 tbsp. unsalted butter
- 2 tbsp. powdered sugar
- 2 cups cold water
- 1 tbsp. sliced cashew

Filling:

- 1 cup shredded coconut
- 2 young coconuts (Remove the flesh)
- 1 cup fresh cream
- 3 tbsp. butter

INSTRUCTIONS

1. Mix the first four ingredients together to create a dough.
2. Roll the batter out into 2 large circles.
3. Press one circle into the pie tin and prick the sides with a fork.
4. Cook the filling ingredients over low heat and pour it in the tin.
5. Cover the pie tin with the second circle.
6. Preheat the fryer to 300 F for 5 minutes.
7. Cook until golden brown, then let it cool.
8. Slice and serve with a dab of cream.

457. Orange Muffins

INGREDIENTS

- 2 cups All-purpose flour
- 1 ½ cup milk
- ½ tsp. baking powder
- ½ tsp. baking soda
- 2 tbsp. butter
- 2 tbsp. sugar
- 2 tsp. vinegar
- 3 tbsp. orange juice and zest
- Muffin cups

INSTRUCTIONS

1. Combine the ingredients except milk to create a crumbly blend.
2. Add this milk to the blend and make a batter and pour into the muffin cups.
3. Preheat the fryer to 300 F and cook 15 minutes.
4. Check whether they are done using a toothpick.

458. Cranberry Cupcakes

INGREDIENTS

- 2 cups All-purpose flour
- 1 ½ cup milk
- ½ tsp. baking powder
- ½ tsp. baking soda
- 2 tbsp. butter
- 2 tbsp. sugar
- 2 tsp. vinegar
- 2 cups grated cranberries
- Muffin cups

INSTRUCTIONS

1. Combine the ingredients except milk to create a crumbly blend.
2. Add this milk to the blend and make a batter and pour into the muffin cups.
3. Preheat the fryer to 300 F and cook 15 minutes.
4. Check whether they are done using a toothpick.

459. Buttermilk and Blueberry Muffins

INGREDIENTS

- 2 cups All-purpose flour
- 1 ½ cup buttermilk
- ½ tsp. baking powder
- ½ tsp. baking soda
- 2 tbsp. butter
- 2 tbsp. sugar
- 2 tsp. vinegar
- 2 cups sliced blueberries
- Muffin cups

INSTRUCTIONS

1. Combine the ingredients except milk to create a crumbly blend.
2. Add this milk to the blend and make a batter and pour into the muffin cups.
3. Preheat the fryer to 300 F and cook 15 minutes.
4. Check whether they are done using a toothpick.

460. Cinnamon Cupcakes

INGREDIENTS

- 2 cups All-purpose flour
- 1 ½ cup milk
- 1 tbsp. cinnamon powder
- ½ tsp. baking powder
- ½ tsp. baking soda
- 2 tbsp. butter
- 2 tbsp. sugar
- Muffin cups

INSTRUCTIONS

1. Combine the ingredients except milk to create a crumbly blend.
2. Add this milk to the blend and make a batter and pour into the muffin cups.
3. Preheat the fryer to 300 F and cook 15 minutes.
4. Check whether they are done using a toothpick.

461. Chocolate Cake

INGREDIENTS

- 1 tbsp. unsalted butter
- 2 tbsp. water
- 2 tbsp. cocoa powder
- 3 tbsp. melted dark chocolate
- 1 cup all-purpose flour
- ½ cup condensed milk

INSTRUCTIONS

1. Add the ingredients together and whisk till you get a smooth mixture.
2. Prepare a tin by greasing it with butter.
3. Transfer the mixture into the tin.
4. Preheat the fryer to 300 F for 5 minutes.
5. You will need to place the tin in the basket and cover it.
6. Check whether the cake has risen well.
7. When the cake has cooled, garnish with chocolate chips and serve.

462. Pumpkin Chocolate Chip Muffins

INGREDIENTS

- 2 cups All-purpose flour
- 1 ½ cup milk
- ½ tsp. baking powder
- ½ tsp. baking soda
- 2 tbsp. butter
- 2 cups grated pumpkin
- 1 tbsp. sugar
- 2 tsp. vinegar
- ½ cup chocolate chips
- Muffin cups

INSTRUCTIONS

1. Combine the ingredients except milk to create a crumbly blend.
2. Add this milk to the blend and make a batter and pour into the muffin cups.
3. Preheat the fryer to 300 F and cook 15 minutes.
4. Check whether they are done using a toothpick.

463. Lemon Poppy Cupcakes

INGREDIENTS

- 2 cups All-purpose flour
- 1 ½ cup milk
- ½ tsp. baking powder
- ½ tsp. baking soda
- 2 tbsp. butter
- 1 tbsp. sugar
- 2 tbsp. lemon juice
- 2 tsp. vinegar
- 1 tbsp. crushed poppy seeds
- Muffin cups

INSTRUCTIONS

1. Combine the ingredients except milk to create a crumbly blend.
2. Add this milk to the blend and make a batter and pour into the muffin cups.
3. Preheat the fryer to 300 F and cook 15 minutes.
4. Check whether they are done using a toothpick.

464. Jalapeño Waffles

INGREDIENTS

- 1 ½ cups almond flour
- 3 eggs
- 2 tsp. dried basil
- 2 tsp. dried parsley
- Salt and Pepper to taste
- 3 tbsp. Butter
- 1 cup pickled Jalapeños

INSTRUCTIONS

1. Preheat the air fryer to 250 F.
2. In a small bowl, mix the ingredients, except the chocolate chips.
3. Take a waffle shape and grease it with butter.
4. Pour the batter and cook till both sides have browned.

465. Corn Muffins

INGREDIENTS

- 2 cups All-purpose flour
- 1 ½ cup milk
- ½ tsp. baking powder
- ½ tsp. baking soda
- 2 tbsp. butter
- 1 tbsp. sugar
- 2 tsp. vinegar
- 1 cup boiled corn
- Muffin cups

INSTRUCTIONS

1. Combine the ingredients except milk to create a crumbly blend.
2. Add this milk to the blend and make a batter and pour into the muffin cups.
3. Preheat the fryer to 300 F and cook 15 minutes.
4. Check whether they are done using a toothpick.

466. Cheddar Muffins

INGREDIENTS

- 2 cups All-purpose flour
- 1 ½ cup milk

- ½ tsp. baking powder
- ½ tsp. baking soda
- 2 tbsp. butter
- 2 cups melted cheddar
- 1 tbsp. sugar
- 2 tsp. vinegar
- Muffin cups

INSTRUCTIONS

1. Combine the ingredients except milk to create a crumbly blend.
2. Add this milk to the blend and make a batter and pour into the muffin cups.
3. Preheat the fryer to 300 F and cook 15 minutes.
4. Check whether they are done using a toothpick.

467.   Honey Banana Muffins

INGREDIENTS

- 2 cups wheat flour
- 1 ½ cup milk
- ½ tsp. baking powder
- ½ tsp. baking soda
- 2 tbsp. butter
- 2 cups mashed banana
- 1 tbsp. honey
- Muffin cups

INSTRUCTIONS

1. Combine the ingredients except milk to create a crumbly blend.
2. Add this milk to the blend and make a batter and pour into the muffin cups.
3. Preheat the fryer to 300 F and cook 15 minutes.
4. Check whether they are done using a toothpick.

468.   Raspberry Buttermilk Cupcakes

INGREDIENTS

- 2 cups All-purpose flour
- 1 ½ cup buttermilk
- ½ tsp. baking powder
- ½ tsp. baking soda
- 2 tbsp. butter

- 2 tbsp. sugar
- 2 cups sliced raspberries
- Muffin cups

INSTRUCTIONS:

1. Combine the ingredients except milk to create a crumbly blend.
2. Add this milk to the blend and make a batter and pour into the muffin cups.
3. Preheat the fryer to 300 F and cook 15 minutes.
4. Check whether they are done using a toothpick.

469.   Vanilla Cake

INGREDIENTS

- 1 tbsp. unsalted butter
- 2 tbsp. water
- 2 tsp. vanilla extract
- 1 cup all-purpose flour
- ½ cup condensed milk

INSTRUCTIONS

1. Add the ingredients together and whisk till you get smooth mixture.
2. Prepare a tin by greasing it with butter. Transfer the mixture into the tin.
3. Preheat the fryer to 300 F for 5 minutes.
4. You will need to place the tin in the basket and cover it.
5. Check whether the cake has risen well.
6. Cool the cake down and serve.

470.   Bacon and Maple Muffins

INGREDIENTS

- 2 cups All-purpose flour
- 1 ½ cup buttermilk
- ½ tsp. baking powder
- ½ tsp. baking soda
- 2 tbsp. butter
- 1 cup finely sliced bacon
- 2 tbsp. maple syrup
- Muffin cups

INSTRUCTIONS

1. Combine the ingredients except milk to create a crumbly blend.
2. Add this milk to the blend and make a batter and pour into the muffin cups.
3. Preheat the fryer to 300 F and cook 15 minutes.
4. Check whether they are done using a toothpick.

471. Butterscotch Muffins

INGREDIENTS

- 2 cups cornstarch
- 1 ½ cup milk
- 3 eggs
- 2 tbsp. butter
- 2 tbsp. sugar
- 1 tsp. vanilla extract
- Muffin cups

INSTRUCTIONS

1. Combine the ingredients except milk to create a crumbly blend.
2. Add this milk to the blend and make a batter and pour into the muffin cups.
3. Preheat the fryer to 300 F and cook 15 minutes.
4. Check whether they are done using a toothpick.

472. Pineapple Pie

INGREDIENTS

- 1 cup plain flour
- 1 tbsp. unsalted butter
- 4tsp. powdered sugar
- 2 cups cold milk

Pineapple filling:

- ½ cup roasted nuts
- 1 pineapple (Peel and chop into slices)
- 2 tbsp. sugar
- ½ tsp. cinnamon
- 2 tsp. lemon juice

INSTRUCTIONS

1. Mix the first four ingredients together to create a dough.
2. Roll the batter out into 2 large circles.
3. Press one circle into the pie tin and prick the sides with a fork.
4. Cook the filling ingredients over low heat and pour it in the tin.
5. Cover the pie tin with the second circle.
6. Preheat the fryer to 300 F for 5 minutes.
7. Cook until golden brown, then let it cool.
8. Slice and serve with a dab of cream.

473. Green citrus Pie

INGREDIENTS

- 1 cup plain flour
- 1 tbsp. unsalted butter
- 4tsp. powdered sugar
- 2 cups cold milk

Filling:

- ½ cup roasted nuts
- 2 tbsp. sugar
- ½ tsp. cinnamon
- 2 tsp. lemon juice
- 4 tsp. lemon zest
- 1 cup sliced kiwi

INSTRUCTIONS

1. Mix the first four ingredients together to create a dough.
2. Roll the batter out into 2 large circles.
3. Press one circle into the pie tin and prick the sides with a fork.
4. Cook the filling ingredients over low heat and pour it in the tin.
5. Cover the pie tin with the second circle.
6. Preheat the fryer to 300 F for 5 minutes.
7. Cook until golden brown, then let it cool.
8. Slice and serve with a dab of cream.

474. Blackberry Pancakes

INGREDIENTS

- 2 - cups minced blackberry
- 1 ½ - cups almond flour

- 3 - eggs
- 2 - tsp. dried basil
- 2 - tsp. dried parsley
- Salt and Pepper to taste
- 3 - tbsp. Butter

INSTRUCTIONS

1. Preheat the air fryer to 250 F.
2. In a small bowl, combine the ingredients. Mix well.
3. Cook till both sides of the pancake have browned.
4. Serve with maple syrup.

475.   Fruit custard

INGREDIENTS

- 1 cup mixed fruits
- 2 cups milk
- 2 tbsp. custard powder
- 3 tbsp. powdered sugar
- 3 tbsp. unsalted butter

INSTRUCTIONS

1. Heat the milk and sugar and add the custard powder, then fruit and mix till you get a thick blend.
2. Preheat the air fryer to 300 F for 5 minutes.
3. Place the dish in the container and lower the temperature to 250 F.
4. Cook for ten minutes and set aside to cool.

476.   Kiwi Custard

INGREDIENTS

- 1 cup kiwi slices
- 2 cups milk
- 2 tbsp. custard powder
- 3 tbsp. powdered sugar
- 3 tbsp. unsalted butter

INSTRUCTIONS

1. Heat the milk and sugar and add the custard powder, then kiwi and mix till you get a thick blend.
2. Preheat the air fryer to 300 F for 5 minutes.

3. Place the dish in the container and lower the temperature to 250 F.
4. Cook for ten minutes and set aside to cool.

477.   Butterscotch Cake

INGREDIENTS

- 1 tbsp. unsalted butter
- 2 tbsp. water
- 2 tsp. vanilla extract
- 2 tbsp. brown sugar
- 1 cup corn flour
- ½ cup condensed milk

INSTRUCTIONS

1. Add the ingredients: together and whisk till you get a smooth mixture.
2. Prepare a tin by greasing it with butter.
3. Transfer the mixture into the tin.
4. Preheat the fryer to 300 F for 5 minutes.
5. You will need to place the tin in the basket and cover it.
6. Check whether the cake has risen well. Cool the cake down and serve.

478.   Cranberry Pudding

INGREDIENTS

- 1 cup cranberry juice
- 2 cups milk
- 2 tbsp. corn flour
- 3 tbsp. powdered sugar
- 3 tbsp. unsalted butter

INSTRUCTIONS

1. Heat the milk and sugar and add the custard powder, then cranberry juice and corn flour and mix till you get a thick blend.
2. Preheat the air fryer to 300 F for 5 minutes.
3. Place the dish in the container and lower the temperature to 250 F.
4. Cook for ten minutes and set aside to cool.

479.   Mediterranean Waffles

INGREDIENTS

- 1 ½ cups almond flour

- 3 eggs
- 2 tsp. dried basil
- 2 tsp. dried parsley
- Salt and Pepper to taste
- 3 tbsp. Butter
- 1 cup coleslaw

INSTRUCTIONS

1. Preheat the air fryer to 250 F.
2. In a small bowl, mix the ingredients, except the coleslaw.
3. Take a waffle shape and grease it with butter.
4. Pour the batter and cook till both sides have browned.
5. Top with coleslaw.

480. Cardamom Cheesecake Muffins

INGREDIENTS

- 2 cups All-purpose flour
- 1 ½ cup milk
- 1 tbsp. cardamom powder
- ½ tsp. baking powder
- 1 cup cheese
- ½ tsp. baking soda
- 2 tbsp. butter
- 2 tbsp. sugar
- Muffin cups

INSTRUCTIONS

1. Combine the ingredients except milk to create a crumbly blend.
2. Add this milk to the blend and make a batter and pour into the muffin cups.
3. Preheat the fryer to 300 F and cook 15 minutes.
4. Check whether they are cone us ng a toothpick.

481. Raspberry Cake

INGREDIENTS

- 1 tbsp. unsalted butter
- 2 tbsp. water
- 2 cups sliced raspberries
- 1 cup all-purpose flour
- ½ cup condensed milk

INSTRUCTIONS

1. Add the ingredients together and whisk till you get a smooth mixture.
2. Prepare a tin by greasing it with butter. Transfer the mixture into the tin.
3. Preheat the fryer to 300 F for 5 minutes.
4. You will need to place the tin in the basket and cover it.
5. Check whether the cake has risen well.
6. When the cake has cooled, garnish with chocolate chips and serve.

482. Dark chocolate Muffins

INGREDIENTS

- 2 cups All-purpose flour
- 1 ½ cup milk
- 3 tbsp. dark cocoa powder
- ½ tsp. baking powder
- ½ tsp. baking soda
- 2 tbsp. butter
- 1 tbsp. sugar
- Muffin cups

INSTRUCTIONS

1. Mix the ingredients together and use your fingers to get a crumbly mixture.
2. Add the baking soda to the milk and mix continuously.
3. Add this milk to the mixture and create a batter, which you will need to transfer to the muffin cups.
4. Preheat the fryer to 300 F for 5 minutes.
5. You will need to place the muffin cups in the basket and cover it.
6. Cook the muffins for 15 minutes and check whether or not the muffins are cooked using a toothpick.
7. Remove the cups and serve hot.

483. Honey and blackberry cake

INGREDIENTS

- 2 cups All-purpose flour
- 1 ½ cup milk
- ½ tsp. baking powder
- ½ tsp. baking soda
- 2 tbsp. butter

- 2 tbsp. honey
- 2 cups sliced blackberry
- 2 tsp. vinegar
- Muffin cups

INSTRUCTIONS

1. Mix the ingredients together and use your fingers to get a crumbly mixture.
2. Add the baking soda and vinegar to the milk and mix continuously.
3. Add this milk to the mixture and create a batter, which you will need to transfer to the muffin cups.
4. Preheat the fryer to 300 F for 5 minutes.
5. You will need to place the muffin cups in the basket and cover it.
6. Cook the muffins for 15 minutes and check whether or not the muffins are cooked using a toothpick.
7. Remove the cups and serve hot.

484. Mexican Waffles

INGREDIENTS

- 1 ½ cups almond flour
- 3 eggs
- 2 tsp. dried basil
- 2 tsp. dried parsley
- Salt and Pepper to taste
- 3 tbsp. Butter
- 1 cup pickled Jalapeños
- 1 cup green olives
- 1 cup black olives
- 2 tbsp. salsa

INSTRUCTIONS

1. Preheat the air fryer to 250 F.
2. In a small bowl, mix the ingredients, except the Jalapeños.
3. Take a waffle shape and grease it with butter. Pour the batter and cook till both sides have browned.
4. Top with Jalapeños.

485. Corn Waffles

INGREDIENTS

- 1 ½ cups almond flour

- 3 eggs
- 2 tsp. dried basil
- 2 tsp. dried parsley
- Salt and Pepper to taste
- 3 tbsp. Butter
- 2 cups boiled corn and mayonnaise

INSTRUCTIONS

1. Preheat the air fryer to 250 F.
2. In a small bowl, mix the ingredients, except the corn and mayo.
3. Take a waffle shape and grease it with butter. Pour the batter and cook till both sides have browned.
4. Top with corn and mayo

486. Blueberry Cake

INGREDIENTS

- 1 tbsp. unsalted butter
- 2 tbsp. water
- 2 cups sliced blueberries
- 1 cup all-purpose flour
- ½ cup condensed milk

INSTRUCTIONS

1. Add the ingredients together and whisk till you get a smooth mixture.
2. Prepare a tin by greasing it with butter. Transfer the mixture into the tin.
3. Preheat the fryer to 300 F for 5 minutes.
4. You will need to place the tin in the basket and cover it.
5. Check whether the cake has risen well.
6. When the cake has cooled, garnish with chocolate chips and serve.

487. Mixed Vegetable Muffins

INGREDIENTS

- 2 cups All-purpose flour
- 1 ½ cup milk
- ½ tsp. baking powder
- ½ tsp. baking soda
- 2 tbsp. butter
- 2 cups mixed vegetables
- 1 tbsp. sugar
- Muffin cups

INSTRUCTIONS

1. Mix the ingredients together and use your fingers to get a crumbly mixture.
2. Add the baking soda to the milk and mix continuously.
3. Add this milk to the mixture and create a batter, which you will need to transfer to the muffin cups.
4. Preheat the fryer to 300 F for 5 minutes.
5. You will need to place the muffin cups in the basket and cover it.
6. Cook the muffins for 15 minutes and check whether or not the muffins are cooked using a toothpick.
7. Remove the cups and serve hot.

488. Vanilla Cupcakes

INGREDIENTS

- 2 cups wheat flour
- 1 ½ cup milk
- ½ tsp. baking powder
- ½ tsp. baking soda
- 2 tbsp. butter
- 1 tbsp. honey
- 3 tbsp. vanilla extract
- 2 tsp. vinegar
- Muffin cups

INSTRUCTIONS

1. Combine the ingredients except milk to create a crumbly blend.
2. Add this milk to the blend and make a batter and pour into the muffin cups.
3. Preheat the fryer to 300 F and cook 15 minutes.
4. Check whether they are done using a toothpick.

489. Pear Muffins

INGREDIENTS

- 2 cups All-purpose flour
- 1 ½ cup buttermilk
- ½ tsp. baking powder
- ½ tsp. baking soda
- 2 tbsp. butter
- 2 tbsp. sugar

- 2 cups sliced pears
- Muffin cups

INSTRUCTIONS:

1. Combine the ingredients except milk to create a crumbly blend.
2. Add this milk to the blend and make a batter and pour into the muffin cups.
3. Preheat the fryer to 300 F and cook 15 minutes.
4. Check whether they are done using a toothpick.

490. Mixed fruit cupcake

INGREDIENTS

- 1 tbsp. unsalted butter
- 2 tbsp. water
- 2 cups mixed fruit
- 1 cup all-purpose flour
- ½ cup condensed milk

INSTRUCTIONS

1. Combine the ingredients except milk to create a crumbly blend.
2. Add this milk to the blend and make a batter and pour into the muffin cups.
3. Preheat the fryer to 300 F and cook 15 minutes.
4. Check whether they are done using a toothpick.

491. Chicken and Honey Muffin

INGREDIENTS

- 2 cups All-purpose flour
- 1 ½ cup buttermilk
- ½ tsp. baking powder
- ½ tsp. baking soda
- 2 tbsp. butter
- 2 cups minced chicken
- 2 tbsp. honey
- Muffin cups

INSTRUCTIONS

1. Combine the ingredients except milk to create a crumbly blend.

2. Add this milk to the blend and make a batter and pour into the muffin cups.
3. Preheat the fryer to 300 F and cook 15 minutes.
4. Check whether they are done using a toothpick.

492. Air Fryer Brownies

Total time: 30 minutes
Servings: 4

INGREDIENTS

Wet:

- 1/4 cup nondairy milk
- 1/4 cup aquafaba
- 1/2 tsp vanilla extract

Dry:

- 1/2 cup whole wheat flour
- 1/2 cup vegan sugar
- 1/4 cup cocoa powder
- 1 tbsp ground flax seeds
- 1/4 tsp salt
- 1/4 cup chopped hazelnuts and mini vegan chocolate chips

INSTRUCTIONS

1. Mix all dry ingredients in a bowl and wet ingredients in a large cup.
2. Add wet and dry together and mix thoroughly.
3. Fold in hazelnuts and chocolate chips.
4. Preheat air fryer to 175° C and line a baking pan with parchment paper.
5. Place the pan in air fryer basket and cook for 20 minutes or until a knife stuck in the middle comes out clean.

493. Air Fryer Carrot Cake in a Mug

Total time: 25 minutes
Servings: 1 cake

INGREDIENTS

- 1 shredded carrot
- 1/4 cup whole wheat flour pastry
- 1 tbsp brown sugar
- 1/4 tsp of baking powder
- 1/4 tsp ground cinnamon

- 2 tbsp and 2 tsp nondairy milk
- 2 tbsp chopped walnuts
- 1 tbsp raisin
- 2 tsp oil
- Pinch of ground allspice
- Pinch of salt

INSTRUCTIONS

1. Oil an oven safe mug
2. Add flour, baking powder, cinnamon, ginger, allspice and salt, and mix together properly with a fork.
3. Add milk, carrots, walnuts, raisins and oil. Mix again.
4. Air fry at 175°C for 15 minutes or until fork inserted into the middle comes out clean.
5. Serve and enjoy.

494. The Heat Wave

INGREDIENTS

- 1 cup plain flour
- 1 tbsp. unsalted butter
- 4tsp. powdered sugar
- 2 cups cold milk

Filling:

- 1 cup sliced pineapple
- 1 cup sliced papaya
- 2 tbsp. sugar
- ½ tsp. cinnamon
- 2 tsp. lemon juice

INSTRUCTIONS

1. Mix the first four ingredients together to create a dough. Roll the batter out into 2 large circles.
2. Press one circle into the pie tin and prick the sides with a fork.
3. Cook the filling ingredients over low heat and pour it in the tin.
4. Cover the pie tin with the second circle.
5. Preheat the fryer to 300 F for 5 minutes.
6. Cook until golden brown, then let it cool.
7. Slice and serve with a dab of cream.

Milton Keynes UK
Ingram Content Group UK Ltd.
UKHW030627050224
437294UK00017B/613